# Advances in the Diagnosis and Management of Uveitis

*Edited by Alejandro Rodriguez-Garcia and C. Stephen Foster*

Published in London, United Kingdom

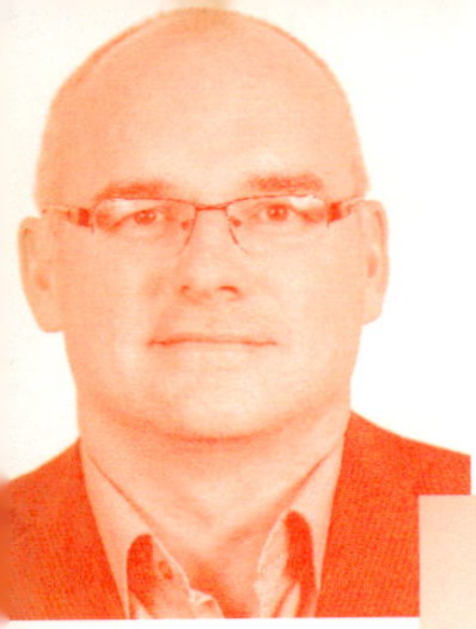
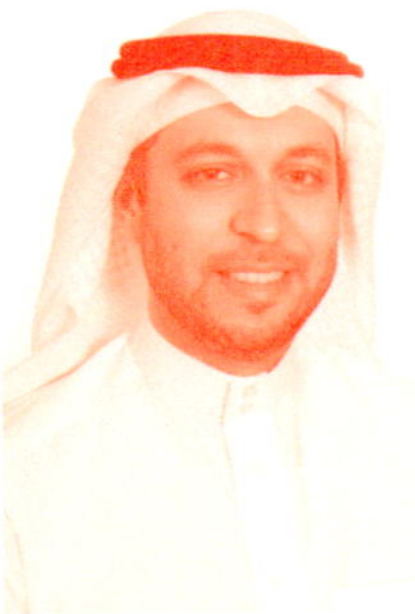
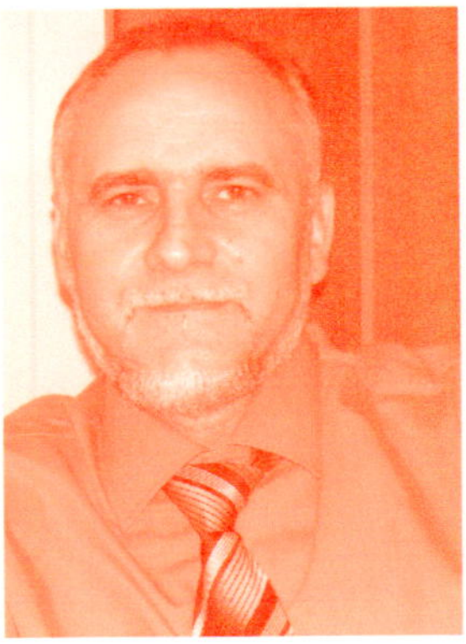
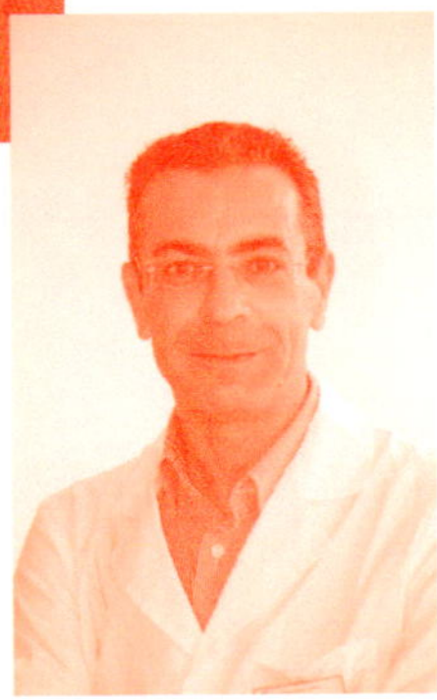
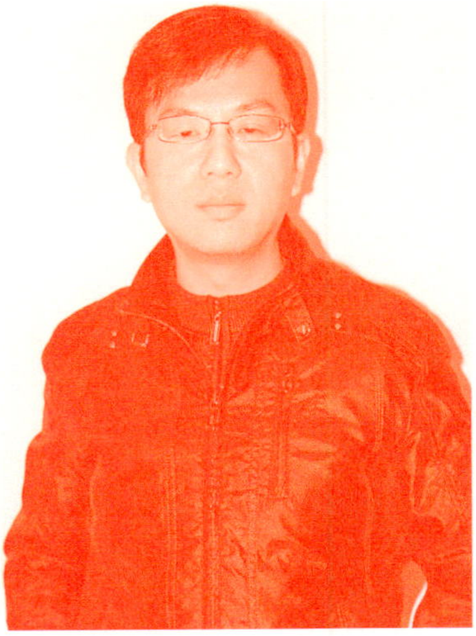
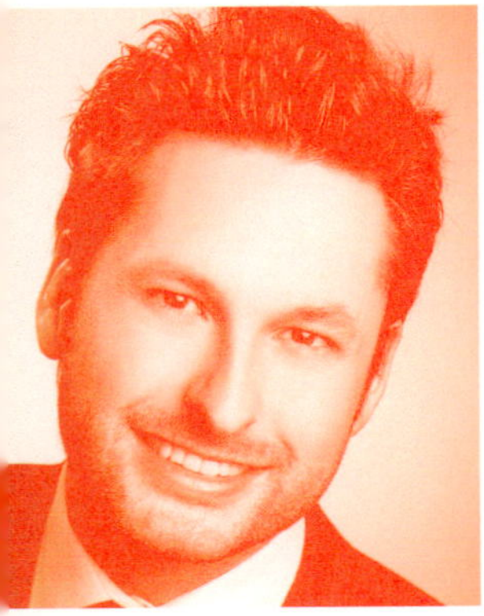
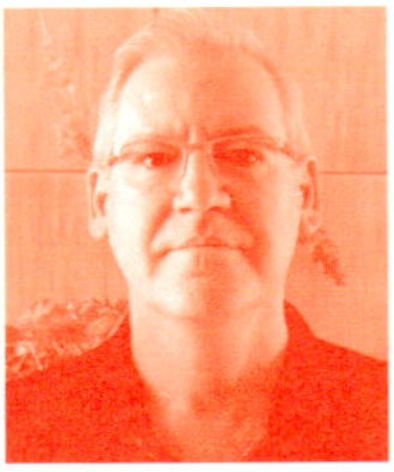

IntechOpen

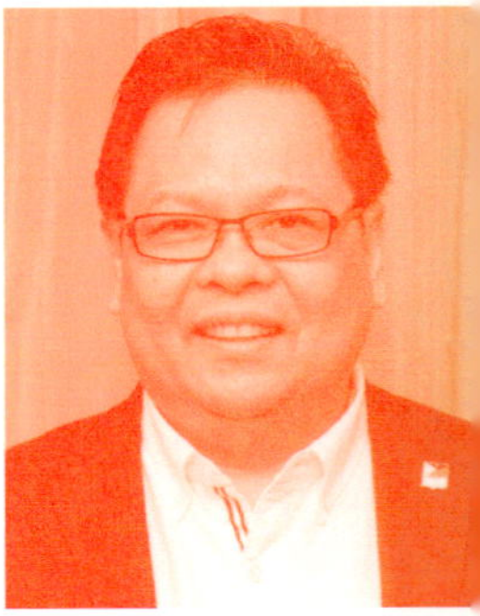
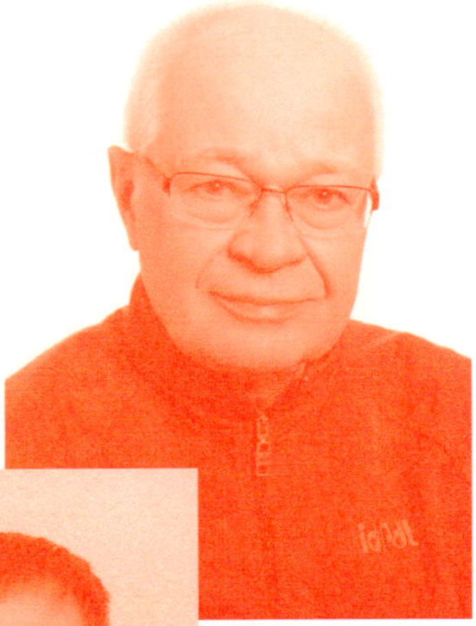
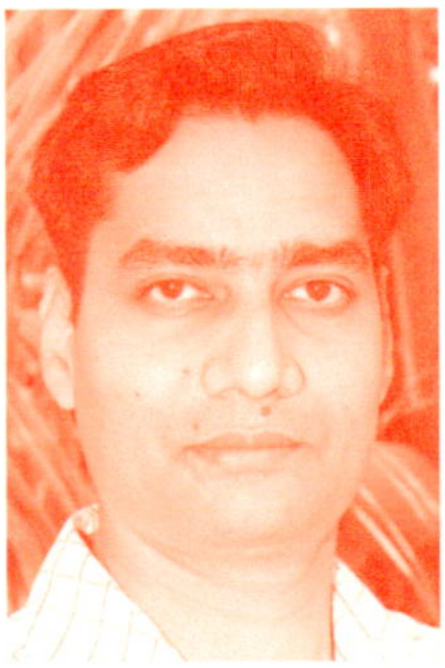
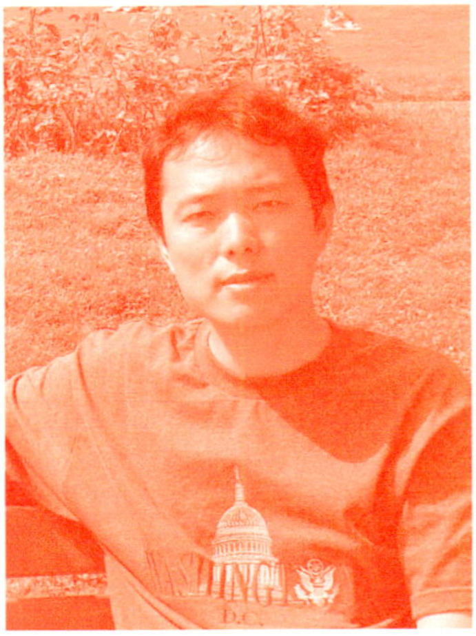
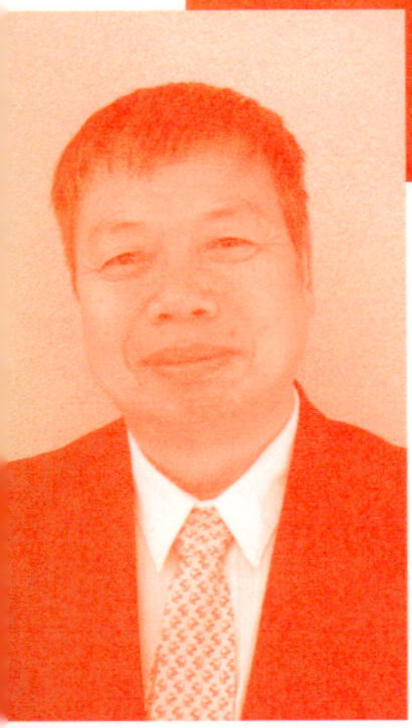
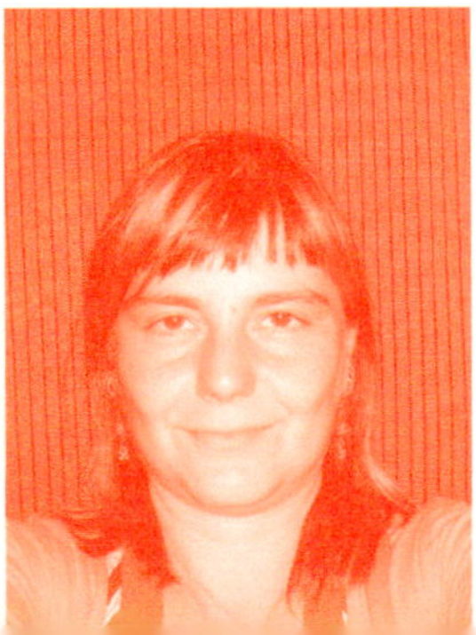

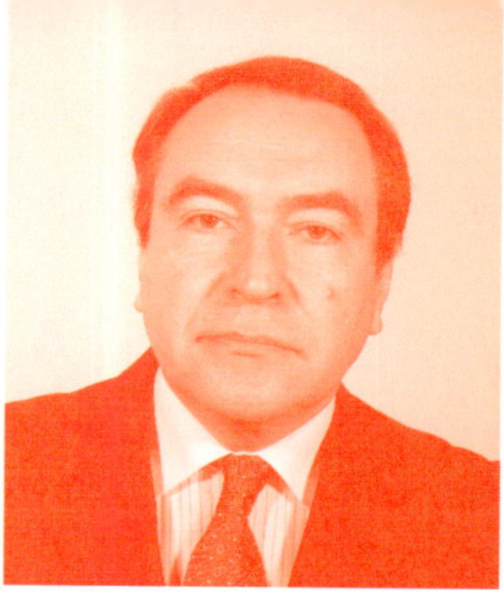
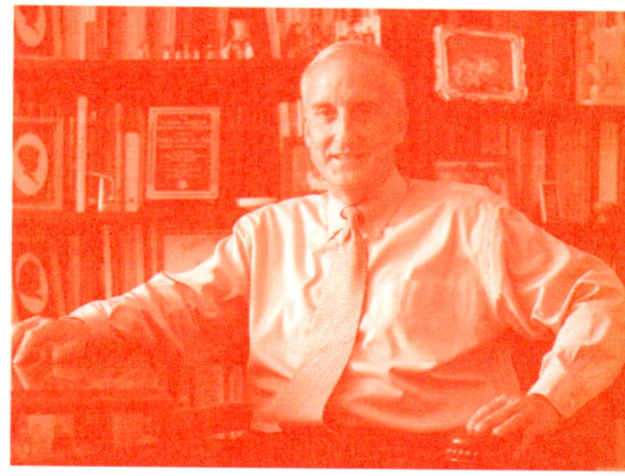
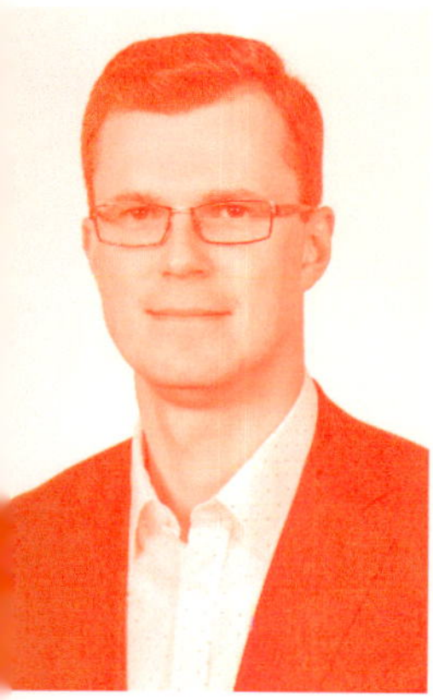
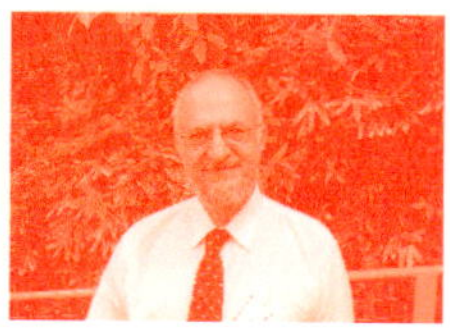
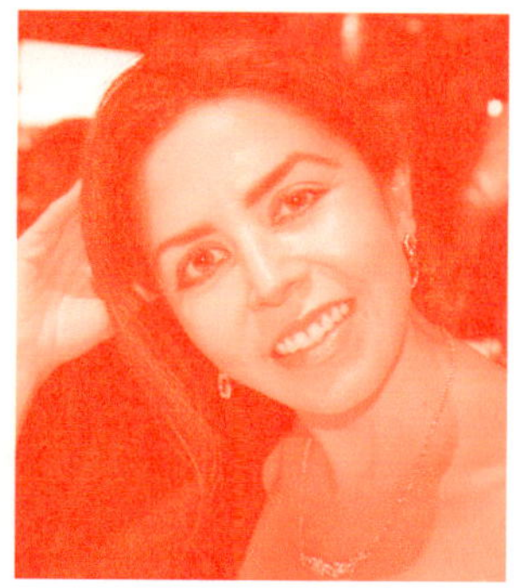

*Supporting open minds since 2005*

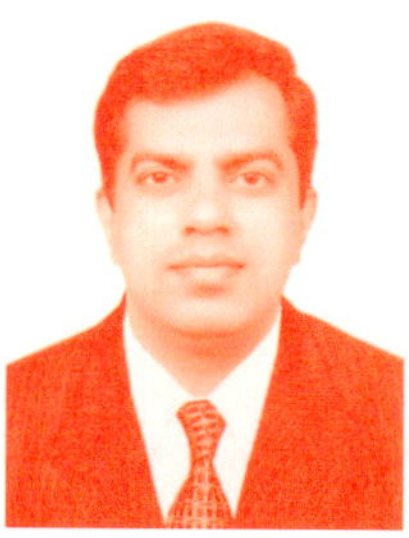
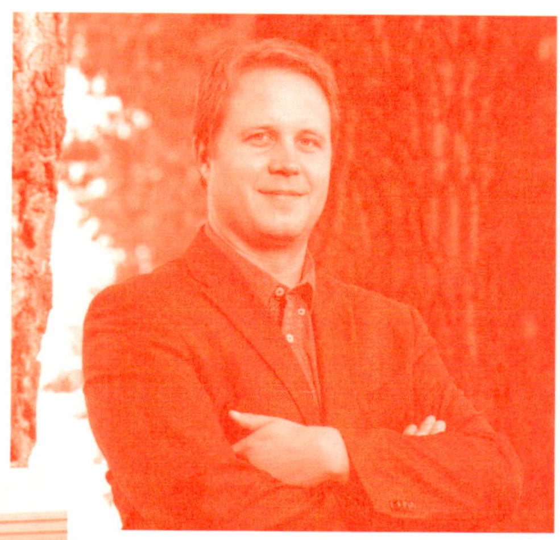
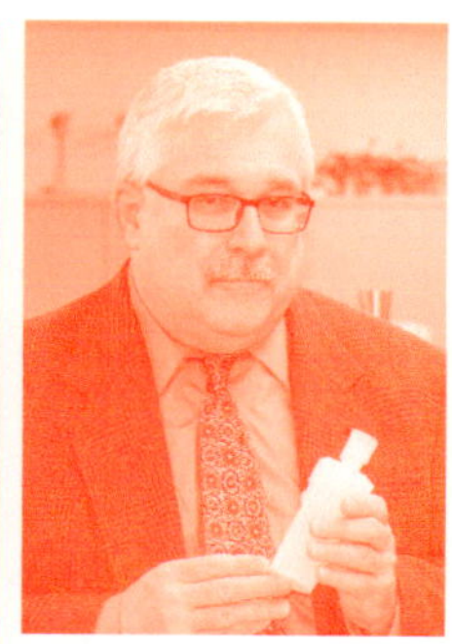
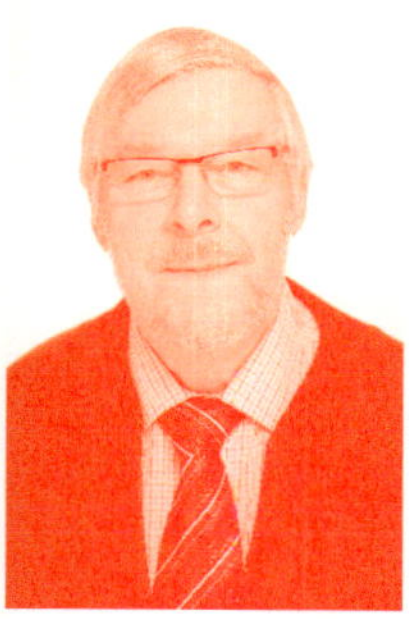
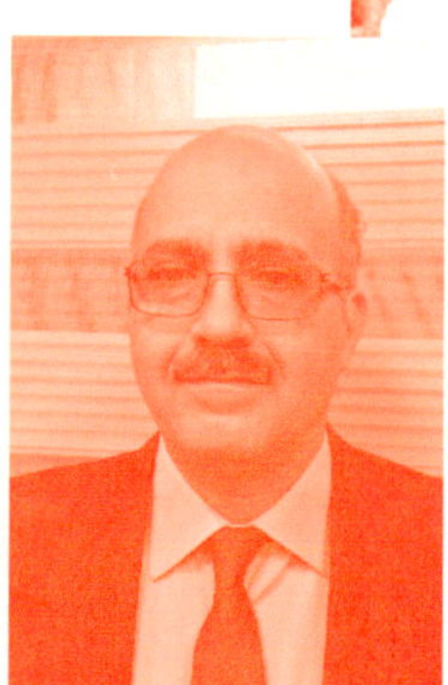
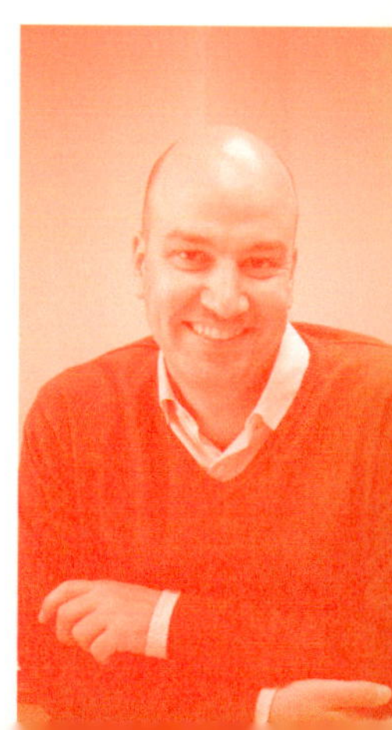
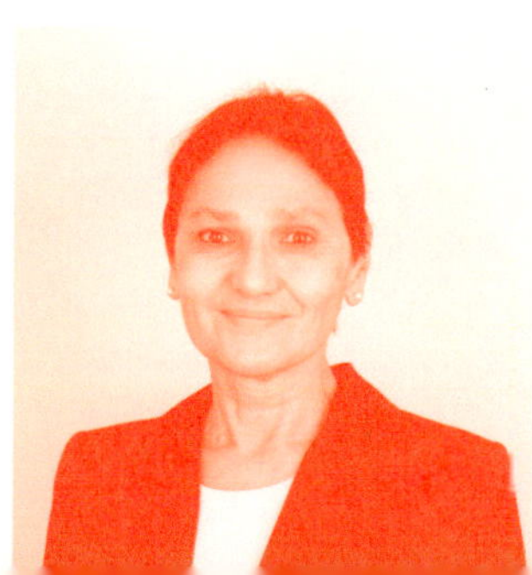

Advances in the Diagnosis and Management of Uveitis
http://dx.doi.org/10.5772/intechopen.73886
Edited by Alejandro Rodriguez-Garcia and C. Stephen Foster

Contributors
Abhinav Dhami, Ravinder Malhi, Darren Lee, Ashvini Reddy, Fauziyya Muhammad, Kongnara Papangkorn, John Higuchi, William Higuchi, Balbir Brar, Cristhian Urzua, Laure Caspers, François Willermain, Dorine Makhoul, Celia Weber, Bahram Bodaghi, Karina Julian, Robison Chan, Pooja Bhat, Ann-Marie Lobo, Judy Chen, Alejandro Rodriguez-Garcia



First published in London, United Kingdom, 2019 by IntechOpen
IntechOpen is the global imprint of INTECHOPEN LIMITED, registered in England and Wales, registration number: 11086078, The Shard, 25th floor, 32 London Bridge Street
London, SE19SG - United Kingdom
Printed in Croatia

British Library Cataloguing-in-Publication Data
A catalogue record for this book is available from the British Library

Additional hard copies can be obtained from orders@intechopen.com

Advances in the Diagnosis and Management of Uveitis
Edited by Alejandro Rodriguez-Garcia and C. Stephen Foster
p. cm.
Print ISBN 978-1-83880-542-5
Online ISBN 978-1-83880-543-2
eBook (PDF) ISBN 978-1-83880-712-2

For EU product safety concerns:
IN TECH d.o.o., Prolaz Marije Krucifikse Kozulić 3, 51000 Rijeka, Croatia, info@intechopen.com or visit our website at intechopen.com.

# Meet the editors

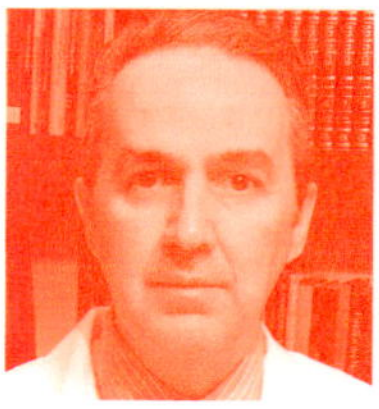

Alejandro Rodriguez-Garcia, MD, is a Clinical and Research Professor of Ophthalmology at Tecnologico de Monterrey School of Medicine & Health Sciences. He is also a Director of the Immunology and Uveitis Service at the Institute of Ophthalmology and Visual Sciences, Zambrano-Hellion Hospital; an Academic and Senior Clinical Research Coordinator of the Multicentric Ophthalmology Residency Program; and a former President of the Center for Ocular Inflammatory Disorders of the Mexican Society of Ophthalmology. Dr. Rodriguez-Garcia received the Best Clinical Professor of Medicine Award. He was appointed as a Professor of Ophthalmology with Best Academic Evaluation, as well as a Postgraduate Professor with the Highest Scientific Production at Tecnologico de Monterrey School of Medicine and Health Sciences. He completed a Clinical and Research Fellowship in Ocular Immunology and Uveitis at the Massachusetts Eye and Ear Infirmary, Harvard Medical School.

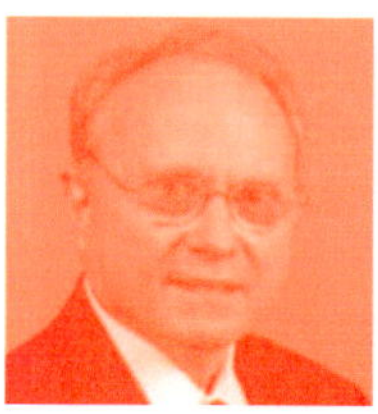

C. Stephen Foster, MD, FAC., FACR, is the Founder and President of the Massachusetts Eye Research and Surgery Institute and the Ocular Immunology and Uveitis Foundation. He is also a Professor of Ophthalmology, part-time, and an Adjunct Professor of Allergy and Immunology, Harvard Medical School; a surgeon in Ophthalmology at the Massachusetts Eye and Ear Infirmary; and a Clinical Associate in Surgery, Massachusetts General Hospital, Harvard Medical School. Dr. Foster received the American Academy of Ophthalmology Award in 1983, the Research to Prevent Blindness Senior Scientific Investigator Award in 1995, and the Mildred Weisenfeld Award for Excellence in Ophthalmology in 2005. He also received a lifetime achievement award from the Academy of Ophthalmology in 2007. In 2016, he was named as one of America's top doctors in ophthalmology for the 15th consecutive year.

# Contents

# Preface

Ocular immunology and uveitis stand as one of the most innovative and developed subspecialties in ophthalmology. Improvements in our understanding of the pathogenic mechanisms, development of more accurate diagnostic tools, and better treatment alternatives for patients with uveitis comes from the continuous efforts of researchers from all over the world who are committed to improving the standard of care of patients suffering from these potentially blinding diseases.

This book focuses on the most recent advances in diagnostic techniques for primary and systemic-associated autoimmune and infectious uveitis, as well as new therapeutic strategies that have significantly reduced the rate of ocular complications and improved the visual outcome of patients suffering from these devastating disorders.

In the introductory chapter, we give an overview of the current diagnostic techniques and therapeutic strategies for uveitis, as well as future trends.

Three sections comprise the book content. The noninfectious uveitis section includes the introductory chapter and two of the most severe forms of chronic panuveitis: Vogt–Koyanagi–Harada (VKH) disease and Behçet's disease. On the one hand, VKH is a common autoimmune disease with a high prevalence among certain ethnic groups, including Hispanics, Asians, and Native Americans; and Behçet's disease is another form of autoimmune vasculitis mainly affecting Asians and Europeans from the Mediterranean basin countries. Both disorders have a prolonged and recurrent clinical course and nowadays continue to represent a vision threat and a therapeutic challenge.

The infectious uveitis section is composed of a chapter on viral retinitis, particularly related to the herpesviruses, one of the most rapidly destructive forms of posterior uveitis. In this chapter, the authors discuss in detail the recent diagnostic tests used for each type of herpesvirus and the specific anti-viral regimens currently used to treat this severe condition. The other chapter from this section focuses on the importance of tuberculosis screening tests to avoid reactivation of latent tuberculosis (TB) related to immunosuppression, particularly with anti-TNFα biologics for patients with different forms of autoimmune uveitis.

The final section of the book focuses on advances in therapeutic strategies for uveitis, covering the therapeutic indications and future perspectives of biologic agents for the management of ocular inflammation. Also, it includes a chapter on an innovative noninvasive intraocular drug delivery system using iontophoresis.

In the future, innovation and development of better diagnostic tools will allow us to increase our diagnostic capability and will reveal many unknown causes of uveitis, closing the gap with the present idiopathic cases. On the other hand, therapeutic strategies should be more specifically targeted and hence more efficient, safer, and better tolerated than present modalities.

We want to thank all the authors involved in this project for their commitment and for sharing their knowledge and expertise in this challenging field that represents uveitis.

**Alejandro Rodriguez-Garcia, MD**
Tecnologico de Monterrey,
School of Medicine and Health Sciences,
Institute of Ophthalmology and Visual Sciences,
Monterrey, Mexico

**C. Stephen Foster, MD, FACS, FACR**
Massachusetts Eye Research and Surgery Institute,
Ocular Immunology and Uveitis Foundation,
Harvard Medical School,
Boston, MA, USA

Section 1

# Noninfectious Uveitis

Chapter 1

# Introductory Chapter: Current and Future Trends in the Diagnosis and Management of Uveitis

*Alejandro Rodriguez-Garcia and C. Stephen Foster*

## 1. Introduction

Uveitis represents a significant burden of visual loss causing around 10–15% of all cases of blindness in the United States, and it is the fifth cause of visual loss in the developed world, accounting for up to 20% of legal blindness [1]. Visual loss due to uveitis currently has a significant impact on the productivity and quality of life of many patients worldwide. Therefore, advances in research and development of diagnostic techniques and therapeutic strategies are crucial for patients suffering from many forms of infectious and autoimmune intraocular inflammation.

One of the main obstacles that ophthalmologists face on diagnosis and treatment of eye disease is the unique complexity of the physical and physiological barriers, as well as the delicate anatomical structures of the human eye. This biologic scenario, particularly in highly destructive tissue disorders like infectious and autoimmune uveitis, represents a challenge for early and accurate diagnosis and effective therapy. Even today, with all possible diagnostic resources available in tertiary eye care facilities, more than 30% of patients suffering from uveitis do not have a definitive etiologic diagnosis [2]. The same is true for current therapeutic methods which suffer from lack of specificity, and are limited to availability at the site of inflammation due to the complex anatomical and physiological characteristics of the eye [3]. Therefore, the development of improved diagnostic methods and therapeutic modalities for inflammatory ocular disorders has recently received special and intense attention by the uveitis research community.

## 2. Advances in diagnosis of uveitis

In the past decades, scientific research at the molecular level and technological development have revolutionized medicine like never before. Such advances, particularly those related to detection technology are significant since early, and accurate diagnosis allows prompt and adequate treatment. Molecular biology has revolutionized medicine with the promise of improving our understanding of the pathogenic mechanisms that produce disease. The human plasma proteome has become the primary target for molecular analysis directed to improve the diagnosis and monitor the therapeutic response of many systemic and ocular disorders. There are at least eight different classes of plasma proteins classified by designed and functional basis. Two such groups are: the "tissue leakage products," which are intracellular proteins that are released into the plasma due to cell damage or death; and the "foreign proteins," which come from infectious microorganisms or parasites



IntechOpen

and are released or exposed to the plasma are the main, but not the only source for diagnostic assays. The plasma proteome has been typically analyzed by electrophoresis combined with chromatography and mass spectrometry [4]. However, many new diagnostic methods have emerged, like DNA microarrays, which may be used for disease diagnosis by detecting biomarkers (genotyping, post-translational modifications, multi-SNPs marker screening, and determination of disease-relevant genes); detecting infectious agents (bacteria, virus, and fungal detection); and genetic disorders (detection of chromosome abnormalities, mutation analysis, and screening of SNPs) [5]. This methodology may interact with other molecular detection methods to study different disease biomarkers from blood, saliva, and other body tissues and fluids like aqueous and vitreous humors. For example, the ability to measure a wide range of molecular components in saliva and compare them to the plasma proteome has become a feasible way to study immunologic markers and microbes for autoimmune and infectious diseases, respectively [6]. Another application of molecular tools like polymerase chain reaction (PCR) has improved the timing for confirmatory diagnosis of infectious uveitis and endophthalmitis [7]. However, the number and type of microorganisms that may be studied in a given sample is limited due to differences in amplification techniques, as well as primers and fluorescent labels availability on multiplex detection systems. More recently, the use of next-generation sequencing (NGS) has proven to be a promising diagnostic strategy for multiple detections of common and rare microorganisms, including virus associated with infectious uveitis and endophthalmitis present in single vitreous samples. An important contribution of NGS so far is related to the improvement of pathogen detection in cases of negative culture endophthalmitis [8].

Despite these promising advances, the development and implementation of many new diagnostic techniques still need to be assessed for their effectiveness regarding precision and accuracy; sensitivity and specificity; predictive value, and cost-benefit balance convenience to be standardized and used widely on a clinical basis.

Imaging diagnostic methods have also suffered significant improvement. The development of the ocular coherence tomography (OCT) which provides non-contact, *in vivo*, cross-sectional, high-speed, and high-resolution images of different ocular structures including the cornea, anterior segment, retina, and optic nerve has evolved from low resolution time-domain image acquisition technology, to spectral domain and swept-source high-definition OCT with en-face, more in-depth, and extended image acquisition modalities [9]. Another significant advancement in diagnostic imaging technology is the development of multimodal devices, which allow the use of different complementary imaging techniques like fluorescein and indocyanine green digital angiography, wide-field angiography, autofluorescence, OCT, and OCT-Angiography all-in-one single machine [10]. Such multimodal equipment has permitted saving costs, time, office space, and less personal rotation when performing multiple studies to a single patient.

Another innovative and very exciting development in ocular image analysis has to do with artificial intelligence (AI), a new field of computer science research that will dramatically change the diagnostic and therapeutic pathways of many chronic degenerative ocular conditions including uveitis. Artificial intelligence already permits early identification of diabetic retinopathy, glaucoma, age-related macular degeneration, retinopathy of prematurity, refractive errors, and cardiovascular risk factors based on color fundus photographs through deep learning algorithms [11]. Very soon, patients will routinely be taken a non-mydriatic fundus photograph at the pre-exam room by an ophthalmic technician allowing the accurate recognition of many systemic associated and primary ocular disorders. Image pattern recognition is the basis of this technology, which requires a large number of fundus photographs to learn from (training dataset) as well as a separate database for validation (validation dataset) [12]. This technology may be coupled with imaging diagnostic devices, such as a fundus camera with fluorescein, indocyanine green, and autofluorescence capabilities; SD-OCT, swept soured OCT, OCT-A, corneal topography, visual system aberrometry and wavefront imaging, anterior segment tomography, and ultrasound, among others, for the detection of specific diagnoses. Soon, this technology will be applied to patients with different forms of uveitis with specific and characteristic clinical appearance analyzed by different image diagnostic devices that will permit the accurate computerized diagnosis in a routine exam.

## 3. Advances in therapy of uveitis

Topical therapy with eye drops makes up more than 90% of ophthalmic formulations including different corticosteroids and non-steroidal anti-inflammatory eye drops. However, their intraocular bioavailability is limited by tear clearance, nasolacrimal drainage, and limited penetration related to the anterior biological barriers including the corneal epithelium and the hemato-aqueous barrier. Moreover, protein binding and enzymatic degradation also account for the limited absorption into target tissues [13]. Many different drug delivery strategies, including prodrugs, chemical permeability enhancers, stimuli-responsive *in situ* gels, and drug delivery carriers like liposomes are being developed to counter the elimination mechanisms mentioned before [14]. The emergence of nanotechnology has impulse the development of such therapeutic strategies for many ocular diseases including uveitis. Different active drugs have been coupled with nanocarriers to overcome the ocular anatomic barriers for direct interaction with specific intraocular tissues, increasing their therapeutic efficiency. Drugs loaded into nanoparticles improve their pharmacodynamics and pharmacokinetics and at the same time, reduce their immunogenicity, biorecognition, and toxicity [15]. One of the most developed fields in ophthalmic pharmacology is the sustained-release intraocular drug delivery devices. Polymeric-controlled release microparticle injections and implants, cyclodextrin-based nanospheres, nanocapsules, microencapsulated cells, liposomes, nano-micelles, and dendrimers are among the most used methods to deliver anti-inflammatory and immunomodulatory drugs into the eye [15, 16]. Such strategies are intended to avoid the side effects of prolonged systemic corticosteroids and immunosuppressive chemotherapy. An intraocular injection may provide a high-dose of medication directly into the site of inflammation with few or no systemic side effects. However, this therapeutic approach is not exempt from potential serious complications like endophthalmitis, vitreous hemorrhage, and retinal detachment, particularly when the administration needs to be repeated several times to achieve their purpose [17]. So far, several polymeric implants are already being used for the control of intraocular inflammation, including corticosteroid formulations [18]. Many other nanotechnology carriers mentioned before may be coupled with different drugs like cyclosporine-A, ganciclovir, non-steroidal anti-inflammatory drugs, anti-angiogenic, and anti-glaucoma medications to be delivered intraocularly. However, because nanoparticles are recently developed, they face several challenges including the need for extensive *in vivo* studies in animal models and then in humans to validate their efficacy and safety. Another essential task is the identification of specific ocular disease-related biomarkers and their cellular and molecular function to develop target-specific drugs that block the biomarker function.

More recently, transscleral iontophoresis has been employed to deliver sufficient dose medications into the eye in a non-invasive way, avoiding injections or the implantation of sustained-release drug devices with minimal side effects [19].

On the other hand, many specific, target-directed biologic molecules manufactured by recombinant DNA technology are used for treating joint systemic and ocular autoimmune inflammation. Such molecules consist of monoclonal antibodies, soluble receptors, cytokines, natural cytokine antagonists, and accessory molecules in antigen presentation. They play critical roles in the pathogenesis of inflammatory uveitis, like TNF-α, IL-1, IL-6; IL-17, T, and B-lymphocytes; and adhesion molecules like LFA-1 and ICAM-1 [20].

Future therapeutic strategies that may be exploited include immune tolerance, inducers of apoptosis, neuroprotective agents, gene therapy, gene transcription factors, and other modulating molecules that permit reprogramming of cells *in vivo*.

## Author details

Alejandro Rodriguez-Garcia[1]* and C. Stephen Foster[2]

1 Tecnologico de Monterrey, School of Medicine and Health Sciences, Institute of Ophthalmology and Visual Sciences, Monterrey, Mexico

2 Massachusetts Eye Research and Surgery Institute, Ocular Immunology and Uveitis Foundation, Harvard Medical School, Boston, MA, USA

*Address all correspondence to: arodri@tec.mx

## References

[1] Durrani OM. Degree, duration, and causes of visual loss in uveitis. British Journal of Ophthalmology. 2004;**88**(9):1159-1162. DOI: 10.1136/bjo.2003.037226

[2] Jabs DA, Nussenblatt RB, Rosenbaum JT. Standardization of Uveitis Nomenclature (SUN) Working Group. Standardization of uveitis nomenclature for reporting clinical data. Results of the First International Workshop. American Journal of Ophthalmology. 2005;**140**(3):509-516

[3] Loftsson T, Sigurdsson HH, Konradsdottir F, Gisladdottir S, Jansook P, Stefansson E. Topical drug delivery to the posterior segment of the eye: Anatomical and physiological considerations. Die Pharmazie - An International Journal of Pharmaceutical Sciences. 2008;**63**(3):171-179. DOI: 10.1691/ph.2008.7322

[4] Anderson NL, Anderson NG. The human plasma proteome. Molecular and Cellular Proteomics. 2002;**1**(11):845-867. DOI: 10.1074/mcp.R200007-MCP200

[5] Yoo SM, Choi JH, Lee SY, Yoo NC. Applications of DNA microarray in disease diagnostics. Journal of Microbiology and Biotechnology. 2008;**19**(7):635-646. DOI: 10.4014/jmb.0803.226

[6] Streckfus CF, Bigler LR. Saliva as a diagnostic fluid. Oral Diseases. 2002;**8**:69-76

[7] Chiquet C, Lina G, Benito Y, Cornut PL, Etienne J, Romanet JP, et al. Polymerase chain identification in aqueous humor of patients with postoperative endophthalmitis. Journal of Cataract and Refractive Surgery. 2007;**33**(4):635-641. DOI: 10.1016/j.jcrs.2006.12.017

[8] Deshmukh D, Joseph J, Chakrabarti M, Sharma S, Jayasudha R, Sama KC, et al. New insights into culture negative endophthalmitis by unbiased next generation sequencing. Scientific Reports. 2019;**9**(1):844. DOI: 10.1038/s41598-018-37502-w

[9] Invernizzi A, Cozzi M, Staurenghi G. Optical coherence tomography and optical coherence tomography angiography in uveitis: A review. Clinical and Experimental Ophthalmology. 2019;**47**(3):357-371. DOI: 10.1111/ceo.13470

[10] Nagiel A, Lalane RA, Sadda SR, Schwartz SD. Ultra-widefield fundus imaging: A review of clinical applications and future trends. Retina. 2016;**36**(4):660-678. DOI: 10.1097/IAE.0000000000000937

[11] Ting D, Cheung C, Lim G, Tan G, Jama NQ. Development and validation of a deep learning system for diabetic retinopathy and related eye diseases using retinal images from multiethnic populations. Journal of the American Medical Association. 2017;**318**(22):2211-2223. DOI: 10.1001/jama.2017.18152

[12] Hogarty DT, Mackey DA, Hewitt AW. Current state and future prospects of artificial intelligence in ophthalmology: A review. Clinical and Experimental Ophthalmology. 2018;**47**(1):128-139. DOI: 10.1111/ceo.13381

[13] Bisht R, Mandal A, Jaiswal JK, Rupenthal ID. Nanocarrier mediated retinal drug delivery: Overcoming ocular barriers to treat posterior eye diseases. Wiley Interdisciplinary Reviews: Nanomedicine and Nanobiotechnology. 2018;**10**(2):e1473. DOI: 10.1002/wnan.1473

[14] Ye T, Yuan K, Zhang W, Song S, Chen F, Yang X, et al. Prodrugs

incorporated into nanotechnology-based drug delivery systems for possible improvement in bioavailability of ocular drugs delivery. Asian Journal of Pharmaceutical Sciences. 2013;**8**(4):207-217. DOI: 10.1016/j.ajps.2013.09.002

[15] Weng Y, Liu J, Jin S, Guo W, Liang X, Hu Z. Nanotechnology-based strategies for treatment of ocular disease. Acta Pharmaceutica Sinica B. 2017;**7**(3):281-291. DOI: 10.1016/j.apsb.2016.09.001

[16] Al-Halafi AM. Nanocarriers of nanotechnology in retinal diseases. Saudi Journal of Ophthalmology. 2014;**28**(4):304-309. DOI: 10.1016/j.sjopt.2014.02.009

[17] Avery RL, Bakri SJ, Blumenkranz MS, Brucker AJ, Cunningham ET Jr, D'Amico DJ, et al. Intravitreal injection technique and monitoring: Updated guidelines of an expert panel. Retina. 2014;**34**(Suppl. 12):S1-S18. DOI: 10.1097/IAE.0000000000000399

[18] Pavesio C, Zierhut M, Bairi K, Comstock TL, Usner DW, Group FAS. Evaluation of an intravitreal fluocinolone acetonide implant versus standard systemic therapy in noninfectious posterior uveitis. Ophthalmology. 2010;**117**(3):567.e1-575.e1. DOI: 10.1016/j.ophtha.2009.11.027

[19] Hastings MS, Li SK, Miller DJ, Bernstein PS, Mufson D. Visulex: Advancing iontophoresis for effective noninvasive back-to-the-eye therapeutics. Drug Delivery Technology. 2004;**4**:53-57

[20] Sharma SM, Fu DJ, Xue K. A review of the landscape of targeted immunomodulatory therapies for non-infectious uveitis. Ophthalmology and therapy. 2018;**7**(1):1-17. DOI: 10.1007/s40123-017-0115-5

Chapter 2

# Vogt-Koyanagi-Harada Disease

*Cristhian A. Urzua*

## Abstract

Vogt-Koyanagi-Harada (VKH) disease is an autoimmune disorder characterized by bilateral intraocular inflammation, exudative retinal detachments, and extraocular manifestations in the auditory, integumentary, and central nervous systems (CNS). This condition is driven by T-cell-mediated autoimmunity directed against melanocytes present in the uveal tissue, in a specific genetic context. The diagnosis is based on clinical presentation, accounting with a set of standardized diagnostic criteria. Studies have reported that patients who have a significant delay in the diagnosis and/or clinical signs of the chronic stage of the disorder have a poorer prognosis and thus special efforts have to be performed in order to have an early diagnosis, together with an appropriate treatment. In that sense, the development of tools that allow us to detect this disease and its degree of severity is extremely important. In this line, novel candidate biomarkers—such as quantification of mRNA levels of NOD and glucocorticoid receptor—have been recently reported, and they represent significant advances that can help the clinician to improve patient categorization and outcomes.

**Keywords:** Vogt-Koyanagi-Harada disease, VKH, vitiligo, treatment response, biomarkers

## 1. Introduction

Vogt-Koyanagi-Harada (VKH) disease is an inflammatory and autoimmune condition characterized by intraocular inflammation, serous retinal detachments, and extraocular manifestations at the level of the auditory, integumentary, and central nervous systems (CNS) [1–3].

No epidemiological studies have been carried out on this condition. However, it has been related to certain geographical areas, such as Latin America and Asia, with a significant contribution of native origin. In this regard, its frequency has been reported up to 22.4% of uveitis causes in referral centers around the world [4–8].

Recently, significant advances have been reported regarding treatment options and novel approaches to evaluate and categorize this group of patients, in order to personalize follow-up and management in each subject and thus achieve better functional and anatomic outcomes [9].

## 2. Pathogenesis

The main disease mechanism would be driven by cell-mediated autoimmunity directed against melanocyte-related proteins, which are located mainly in the uveal tissue, skin, and CNS. A significant body of evidence has been published regarding the role of genetic associations. The human leukocyte antigen (HLA) appears as a risk factor for VKH, and particularly HLA-DR alleles have shown more consistent data [10, 11]. Moreover, several associations with certain polymorphisms have been reported in Chinese population. In this regard, important advances regarding the role of genetic background in VKH have been introduced by Yang et al. This group has been extensively studying different polymorphisms in VKH in Chinese population [12].

Regarding the role of the immune system in VKH pathogenesis, CD4 + lymphocytes and key cytokines—such as interleukin-2 and interferon gamma—appear to play central roles in the development of autoimmunity against melanocyte-associated proteins [13–15].

## 3. Clinical findings

A prodromal stage may precede the ocular involvement. This stage is characterized by tinnitus and meningismus, which may include nausea, vomiting, stiffness of the neck and back, as well as headache as a frequent symptom. However, despite its high frequency, headache cannot be considered as a sufficient criterion for the definition of meningismus. By this stage, if lumbar puncture is performed, it may be returned with pleocytosis [3, 16].

After this prodromal phase of neurological findings, the disease continues toward ocular involvement, presenting bilateral acute panuveitis, with a low grade of anterior chamber cells and vitreous haze, and diffuse choroiditis, associated with exudative retinal detachments and optic disc swelling [1, 16–18] (**Figure 1**).

Following this initial uveitic phase, a significant group of patients may develop chronic granulomatous inflammation, and progressive depigmentation of the fundus resulting in "sunset glow fundus" appearance and/or chorioretinal atrophy (**Figure 2**). These clinical findings frequently result from insufficiently treated or from a late diagnosis, and they have been associated with poorer functional outcomes [19–21].

Experimental studies have reported choroidal infiltration of activated lymphocytes in patients with "sunset glow fundus," suggesting a persistent low grade of subclinical inflammation, which may be implicated in the mechanism of autoimmune-mediated ocular depigmentation and atrophy [22, 23].

In addition, integumentary findings may be seen in some patients. In this regard, alopecia, poliosis, and vitiligo are classic signs related to pathological autoimmune response directed to pigmented tissues (**Figure 3**).

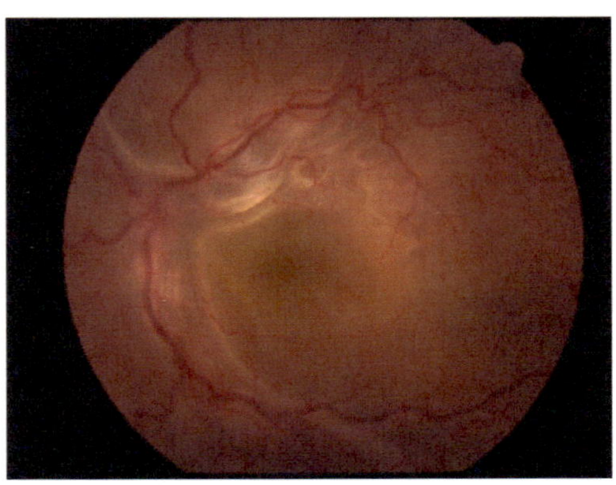

**Figure 1.**
*Color fundus photo showing extensive areas of subretinal fluid and bullous serous retinal detachment in a 37-year-old female with VKH.*

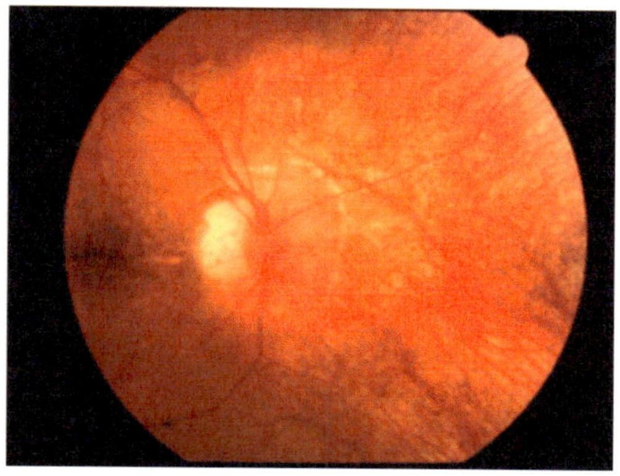

**Figure 2.**
*Extensive fundus depigmentation in a VKH patient after 1 year of disease onset. Note the characteristic "sunset glow" appearance of the fundus.*

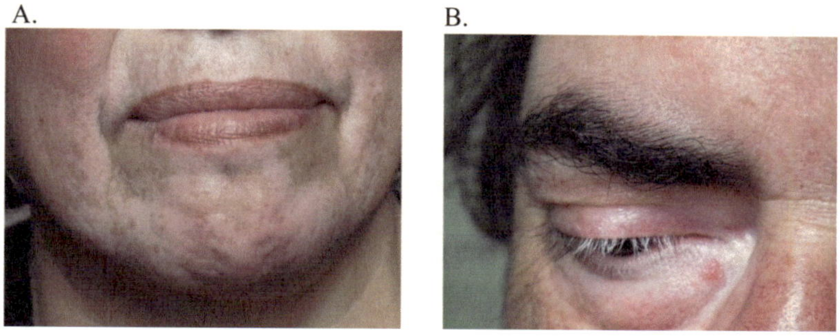


**Figure 3.**
*Integumentary findings in VKH patients. (A) Areas of vitiligo in the perioral area and (B) poliosis in two adult patients with VKH.*

## 4. Diagnosis

Diagnosis of VKH involves a comprehensive ophthalmic evaluation, in order to confirm the presentation of characteristic findings described above. Importantly, the bilateral nature of the condition and the presence of panuveitis, with areas of subretinal fluid and/or retinal detachments, as well as the inexistence of evidence of alternative diseases are hallmarks of the set of standardized diagnostic criteria previously published (**Table 1**) [3, 9, 24]. In that sense, the presence of integumentary and/or neurological findings defines the category of diagnosis (probable

| |
|---|
| 1. No previous history of penetrating ocular trauma or surgery |
| 2. No clinical/laboratory evidence suggestive of another ocular condition |
| 3. **Ocular findings**: bilateral ocular involvement (*a or b must be present*): |
| a. Early manifestations: |
| a.1. Diffuse choroiditis, which may manifest as one of the following: focal areas of subretinal fluid and bullous serous retinal detachment |
| a.2. With equivocal fundus findings, both of the following must be present: characteristic *fluorescein retinal angiogram* findings (focal areas of delay on choroidal perfusion, multifocal areas of pinpoint leakage, large placoid areas of hyperfluorescence, pooling within subretinal fluid, optic nerve staining) and diffuse choroidal thickening without evidence of posterior scleritis on *ultrasonography* |

| |
|---|
| b. Late manifestations: |
| b.1. History suggestive of prior presence of early manifestations and either both b.2 and b.3 findings or multiple signs from b.3 |
| b.2. Ocular depigmentation (either of the following is sufficient): sunset glow fundus or Sugiura sign |
| b.3. Other ocular signs: nummular chorioretinal scars, retinal pigment epithelium clumping and/or migration, or recurrent/chronic anterior uveitis |
| 4. **Neurological/auditory findings**: |
| a. Meningismus |
| b. Tinnitus |
| c. Pleocytosis on cerebrospinal fluid |
| 5. **Integumentary findings** (not preceding ocular and neurological involvement): |
| a. Alopecia |
| b. Poliosis |
| c. Vitiligo |
| Diagnostic categories (*criteria 1 and 2 must be always present*): |
| 1. Complete: ocular plus neurological/auditory plus integumentary findings |
| 2. Incomplete: ocular plus either neurological/auditory or integumentary findings |
| 3. Probable: only ocular findings |
| **Modified from Read et al. [3].* |

**Table 1.**
*Revised diagnostic criteria for Vogt-Koyanagi-Harada disease*.*

if only ocular findings are found, incomplete if at least an extraocular criteria is documented, and complete if all the extraocular criteria may be found) [3, 4, 25].

Despite these previously published diagnostic criteria, a moderate agreement among uveitis experts has been recently reported for the diagnosis of VKH, with a calculated kappa coefficient of 0.4 [25].

## 5. Treatment

The cornerstone of the therapy corresponds to the use of systemic corticosteroids (CS), based on the following principles: early treatment initiation, intensive (initial dose of prednisolone/prednisone of 1 mg/kg/day, with a maximum dose of 80 mg/day), and prolonged (at least 6 months) [27, 28].

Despite this aggressive therapy with systemic CS, a significant proportion of VKH patients present refractoriness, remaining with active inflammation and thus requiring immunomodulatory therapy (IMT) [9]. This subset of refractory patients has better functional outcomes if an earlier IMT is indicated [9].

Therefore, an early CS-response categorization should be carried out, in order to distinguish and to separate subjects with a potential benefit of early IMT initiation. In that sense, some clinical predictive factors of GC refractoriness have been described, such as baseline VA $\leq$ 20/200, fundus depigmentation at diagnosis, and chronic disease, which are important facts to be considered in the context of an appropriate VKH initial evaluation [9].

Currently, a trend to the use of IMT, as first-line therapy, has been observed, with no preference in terms of a specific immunosuppressant [29].

## 6. Novel biomarkers of treatment response and disease activity

As stated above, systemic CS play a significant role for the management of VKH patients. CS have been broadly used for autoimmune and inflammatory diseases. It is a family of lipophilic medications that has its main mechanism of action at the level of the cellular nucleus, interacting directly with the DNA, enhancing or repressing gene expression [30].

Some significant developments have been published regarding potential biomarkers of treatment response based on the glucocorticoid receptor (GR), which is a ligand-dependent transcriptional factor [30]. Urzua et al. have found a distinct expression profile of GR isoforms that allows to categorize GC response as early as 2 weeks [26]. This laboratory-based approach is based on the quantification of mRNA levels of GR isoforms in two time points and a ratio calculation between both measurements. Furthermore, an in vitro assay has been developed, using a similar strategy based on GR expression measurements after in vitro manipulation of immune cells of VKH patients. In that sense, a single blood sample is required, and patient compliance is not mandatory since sampling for a second time or a CS systemic therapy is not required to perform the experiments (Urzua et al., data not published).

As previously described VKH may present with episodes of subclinical inflammation in which, despite clinical examination may appear with no disease activity, there is evidence of inflammatory foci at the level of choroid, using ancillary testing [17]. Although there have been efforts to standardize clinical examination in patients with uveitis, some issues remain, mainly related to the accuracy of measurements and subjectivity, especially with the clinical quantification of flare and vitreous inflammation [31, 32]. In that sense, a novel laboratory-based tool to categorize disease activity in VKH patients has been recently initiated. Following previous reports regarding the utility of GR quantification to evaluate treatment response in VKH, a protein implicated in this pathway has been studied as a candidate biomarker. A phosphatase of the MAPK pathway has been evaluated in different in vitro experimental conditions, and it has been found to have an association between its expression profile and disease activity in VKH patients (Urzua et al., data not published).

Significant evidence has been published regarding potential biomarkers for disease activity. In that sense, Yang et al. have reported a higher expression of NOD1/NOD2 and osteopontin (a matricellular protein) in patients with active VKH in comparison with healthy controls and inactive VKH [33, 34].

These promising biomarkers may help clinicians to make decisions in an inflammatory condition, which can present with significant choroidal inflammation with the absence of clinical evidence of active inflammation, with a resulting worsening in prognosis, in terms of sunset glow fundus and visual outcomes [21].

## Author details

Cristhian A. Urzua[1,2]

1 Facultad de Medicina, Clinica Alemana-Universidad del Desarrollo, Santiago, Chile

2 Laboratorio de Enfermedades Autoinmunes Oculares y Sistemicas, Facultad de Medicina, Universidad de Chil, Santiago, Chile

*Address all correspondence to: cristhian.urzua@uchile.cl

## References

[1] Moorthy RS, Inomata H, Rao NA. Vogt-Koyanagi-Harada syndrome. Survey of Ophthalmology. 1995;**39**:265-292

[2] Read RW, Rao NA. Utility of existing Vogt-Koyanagi-Harada syndrome diagnostic criteria at initial evaluation of the individual patient: a retrospective analysis. Ocular Immunology and Inflammation. 2000;**8**:227-234

[3] Read RW, Holland GN, Rao NA, et al. Revised diagnostic criteria for Vogt-Koyanagi-Harada disease: report of an international committee on nomenclature. American Journal of Ophthalmology. 2001;**131**:647-652

[4] Greco A, Fusconi M, Gallo A, et al. Vogt-Koyanagi-Harada syndrome. Autoimmunity Reviews. 2013;**12**:1033-1038

[5] Kim MH, Seong MC, Kwak NH, et al. Association of HLA with Vogt-Koyanagi-Harada syndrome in Koreans. American Journal of Ophthalmology. 2000;**129**:173-177

[6] Liberman P, Gauro F, Berger O, Urzua CA. Causes of Uveitis in a tertiary center in Chile: A cross-sectional retrospective review. Ocular Immunology and Inflammation. 2015;**23**:339-345

[7] Nguyen M, Siak J, Chee SP, Diem VQH. The spectrum of Uveitis in Southern Vietnam. Ocular Immunology and Inflammation. 2017;**25**:S100-S106

[8] Yang P, Ren Y, Li B, Fang W, Meng Q, Kijlstra A. Clinical characteristics of Vogt-Koyanagi-Harada syndrome in Chinese patients. Ophthalmology. 2007;**114**:606-614

[9] Urzua CA, Velasquez V, Sabat P, et al. Earlier immunomodulatory treatment is associated with better visual outcomes in a subset of patients with Vogt-Koyanagi-Harada disease. Acta Ophthalmologica. 2015;**93**:e475-e480

[10] Weisz JM, Holland GN, Roer LN, et al. Association between Vogt-Koyanagi-Harada syndrome and HLA-DR1 and -DR4 in Hispanic patients living in southern California. Ophthalmology. 1195;**102**:1012-1015

[11] Arellanes-Garcia L, Bautista N, Mora P, et al. HLA-DR is strongly associated with Vogt-Koyanagi-Harada disease in Mexican Mestizo patients. Ocular Immunology and Inflammation. 1998;**6**:93-100

[12] Ng JY, Luk FO, Lai TY, Pang CP. Influence of molecular genetics in Vogt-Koyanagi-Harada disease. Journal of Ophthalmic Inflammation and Infection. 2014;**4**:20

[13] Hou S, Du L, Lei B, et al. Genome-wide association analysis of Vogt-Koyanagi-Harada syndrome identifies two new susceptibility loci at 1p31.2 and 10q21.3. Nature Genetics. 2014;**46**:1007-1011

[14] Silpa-Archa S, Silpa-Archa N, Preble JM, Foster CS. Vogt-Koyanagi-Harada syndrome: Perspectives for immunogenetics, multimodal imaging, and therapeutic options. Autoimmunity Reviews. 2016;**15**:809-819

[15] Sugita S, Takase H, Taguchi C, et al. Ocular infiltrating CD4+ T cells from patients with Vogt-Koyanagi-Harada disease recognize human melanocyte antigens. Investigative Ophthalmology & Visual Science. 2006;**47**:2547-2554

[16] Attia S, Khochtali S, Kahloun R, Zaouali S, Khairallah M. Vogt–Koyanagi–Harada disease. Expert Review of Ophthalmology. 2012;**7**:565-585

[17] Bouchenaki N, Cimino L, Auer C, Tao Tran V, Herbort CP. Assessment

and classification of choroidal vasculitis in posterior uveitis using indocyanine green angiography. Klinische Monatsblätter für Augenheilkunde. 2002;**219**:243-249

[18] Bouchenaki N, Herbort CP. Stromal choroiditis. In: Pleyer UMB, editor. Essentials in Ophthalmology: Uveitis and Immunological Disorders. Berlin, Heidelberg, New York: Springer; 2004. pp. 234-253

[19] Abu El-Asrar AM, Al Tamimi M, Hemachandran S, Al-Mezaine HS, Al-Muammar A, Kangave D. Prognostic factors for clinical outcomes in patients with Vogt-Koyanagi-Harada disease treated with high-dose corticosteroids. Acta Ophthalmologica. 2013;**91**:e486-e493

[20] Abu El-Asrar AM, Al Mudhaiyan T, Al Najashi AA, et al. Chronic recurrent Vogt-Koyanagi-Harada disease and development of 'Sunset Glow Fundus' predict worse retinal sensitivity. Ocular Immunology and Inflammation. 2017;**25**:475-485

[21] Kawaguchi T, Horie S, Bouchenaki N, Ohno-Matsui K, Mochizuki M, Herbort CP. Suboptimal therapy controls clinically apparent disease but not subclinical progression of Vogt-Koyanagi-Harada disease. International Ophthalmology. 2010;**30**:41-50

[22] Inomata H, Sakamoto T. Immunohistochemical studies of Vogt-Koyanagi-Harada disease with sunset sky fundus. Current Eye Research 9 Suppl:35-40, 1990

[23] Bacsal K, Wen DS, Chee SP. Concomitant choroidal inflammation during anterior segment recurrence in Vogt-Koyanagi-Harada disease. American Journal of Ophthalmology. 2008;**145**:480-486

[24] da Silva FT, Damico FM, Marin ML, et al. Revised diagnostic criteria for vogt-koyanagi-harada disease: considerations on the different disease categories. American Journal of Ophthalmology. 2009;**147**:339-345.e5

[25] Jabs DA, Dick A, Doucette JT, et al. Interobserver Agreement Among Uveitis Experts on Uveitic Diagnoses: The Standardization of Uveitis Nomenclature Experience. American Journal of Ophthalmology. 2018;**186**:19-24

[26] Urzua CA, Guerrero J, Gatica H, Velasquez V, Goecke A. Evaluation of the Glucocorticoid Receptor as a Biomarker of Treatment Response in Vogt-Koyanagi-Harada Disease. Investigative Ophthalmology & Visual Science. 2017;**58**:974-980

[27] Nazari H, Rao NA. Resolution of subretinal fluid with systemic corticosteroid treatment in acute Vogt-Koyanagi-Harada disease. The British Journal of Ophthalmology. 2012;**96**:1410-1414

[28] Read RW, Yu F, Accorinti M, et al. Evaluation of the effect on outcomes of the route of administration of corticosteroids in acute Vogt-Koyanagi-Harada disease. American Journal of Ophthalmology. 2006;**142**:119-124

[29] Paredes I, Ahmed M, Foster CS. Immunomodulatory therapy for Vogt-Koyanagi-Harada patients as first-line therapy. Ocular Immunology and Inflammation. 2006;**14**:87-90

[30] Truss M, Beato M. Steroid hormone receptors: Interaction with deoxyribonucleic acid and transcription factors. Endocrine Reviews. 1993;**14**:459-479

[31] Denniston AK, Holland GN, Kidess A, et al. Heterogeneity of primary outcome measures used in clinical trials of treatments for intermediate, posterior, and panuveitis. Orphanet Journal of Rare Diseases. 2015;**10**:97

[32] Kempen JH, Ganesh SK, Sangwan VS, Rathinam SR. Interobserver agreement in grading activity and site of inflammation in eyes of patients with uveitis. American Journal of Ophthalmology. 2008;**146**:813-818.e1

[33] Chu M, Yang P, Hu R, et al. Elevated serum osteopontin levels and genetic polymorphisms of osteopontin are associated with Vogt-Koyanagi-Harada disease. Investigative Ophthalmology & Visual Science. 2011;**52**:7084-7089

[34] Deng B, Ye Z, Li L, et al. Higher expression of NOD1 and NOD2 is associated with Vogt-Koyanagi-Harada (VKH) syndrome but not behcet's disease (BD). Current Molecular Medicine. 2016;**16**:424-435

Chapter 3

# Behcet's Disease

*Karina Julian and Bahram Bodaghi*

## Abstract

Defined as a systemic vasculitis developing in a particular genetic background, uveitis is one of the hallmarks to diagnose Behcet's disease and also one of the important clinical criteria to start systemic treatment. Isolated anterior non granulomatous uveitis with hypopyon, even though a classic clinical picture, actually develops in a minority of cases. In most patients, uveitis is posterior, associated to small vessel occlusive retinal vasculitis, carrying a high risk of permanent retinal damage and subsequent severe visual loss. The guarded natural prognosis of the disease has positively changed in the last decennials with the introduction of biologic immunosuppressant agents in the field of uveitis. Vision can be preserved in most cases provided a prompt early diagnosis and adequate therapy. The potential role of oral bacteria as a triggering factor for autoinflammation in predisposed hosts is interesting, opening the door to prevention in this still not well-understood severe uveitis.

**Keywords:** hypopyon uveitis, occlusive vasculitis, retinitis, retinal atrophy, immunosuppressants

## 1. Introduction

Named after the Turkish ophthalmologist, Hulusi Behcet (who described in 1937 the classic triad of oral aphthosis, genital ulcers, and hypopyon uveitis) [1], Behcet's disease (BD) is a systemic relapsing obliterative vasculitis, affecting arteries, veins, and mainly capillaries. Even though almost all organs can eventually be involved, the compromise of the central nervous system (CNS) and eye makes the disease's prognosis guarded and usually urges to start proper treatment.

There is no specific test to diagnose Behcet's disease: by definition, its diagnosis is a clinical one. In 1990, the International Study Group for Behcet's disease established a set of diagnostic criteria in an attempt to unify the five different ones used by that time [2]. They required the presence of oral ulcerations plus any two of genital ulcerations, typical defined eye lesions, typical defined skin lesions or a positive pathergy test.

Far from being solved, the debate on the diagnostic criteria is still active, and many other sets have been proposed. Among them, the Behcet's Disease Research Committee of Japan defines the diagnosis as complete or incomplete upon the presence of major and minor symptoms (**Table 1**) [3]. The Dilsen criteria (revised in 2000) seems more suitable to the European patients suffering from Behcet's disease (**Table 2**) [4, 5].

| |
|---|
| 1. Major symptoms |
| (a) Recurrent aphthous oral ulcers |
| (b) Skin lesions: erythema nodosum-like lesions, thrombophlebitis, folliculitis, and cutaneous hypersensitivity |
| (c) Ocular symptoms: iridocyclitis, retinitis, and sequelae of uveitis |
| (d) Genital ulcers |
| 2. Minor symptoms |
| (a) Arthritis |
| (b) Intestinal Behcet's disease |
| (c) Epididymitis |
| (d) Vascular lesions |
| (e) Neurologic lesions |
| 3. Examination |
| Pathergy test |
| 4. Diagnosis |
| A. Complete type: all four major symptoms present |
| B. Incomplete type:<br>• Three major symptoms present<br>• Two major and two minor symptoms present<br>• Ocular symptoms and one other major symptom present<br>• Ocular symptoms and two minor symptoms present |

**Table 1.**
*Behcet's Disease Research Committee of Japan: diagnostic criteria.*

| |
|---|
| Three out of the five following criteria are required to diagnose Behcet's disease |
| 1. Recurrent oral ulcers |
| 2. Recurrent genital ulcers |
| 3. Skin lesions |
| 4. Eye lesions |
| 5. Thrombophlebitis |
| (+) Skin pathergy test |
| Always exclude other causative factors |

**Table 2.**
*Behcet's disease: the Dilsen criteria.*

## 2. Clinical picture

### 2.1 Non-ocular disease

Almost every organ and system can eventually be affected by this severe vasculitis. Painful, recurrent oral and genital ulcers are so frequent that their presence is part of the diagnostic criteria [6]. Other skin manifestations are papulopustules, acneiform dermatitis, and erythema nodosum [7]. Arthritis is also a common manifestation of the disease [8]. Gastrointestinal involvement affects around 3–30% of cases with symptoms overlapping inflammatory bowel disease [9]. Central nervous system (CNS) involvement can touch almost 31% of patients and makes the prognosis guarded [10]. Venous thrombosis and arterial aneurysms are present in around 25% of cases [11].

### 2.2 Ocular disease

The classic clinical picture is the one of recurrent, bilateral, non-granulomatous posterior or panuveitis with retinal vasculitis. This is the case for almost 80% of patients, while in around 10% disease manifests as anterior, non-granulomatous uveitis with hypopyon and eventually synechiae (**Figure 1**) [12].

Disease seems to be more severe in males, and ocular pain, redness, photophobia, and blurred vision are almost always present.

Retinitis is also a classic and sight-threatening manifestation of posterior segment involvement, leading most of the time to retinal atrophy. Indeed, Behcet's disease is one of the differential diagnoses of macular atrophy related to uveitis (**Figure 2**) [13].

Retinal vasculitis is the hallmark of the disease, it is obliterative in nature, it affects both arteries and veins, and, most importantly, it involves the capillaries [14].

Behcet's disease is mainly a capillaropathy, being fluorescein angiography (FA) essential to its proper diagnosis and management. FA will better delineate areas of non-perfusion (**Figure 3**), capillary leakage (**Figure 4**), and vascular remodeling. The "fern-leaf"-shaped leakage pattern from capillaries, even though not pathognomonic, is highly evocative of BD (**Figure 5**).

Given the highly vascularized nature of choroidal tissue, it is not surprising to see choroidal involvement during active disease. Indocyanine green angiography (ICGA) shows irregular filling of the choriocapillaris, choroidal filling defects, and dye leakage from choroidal vessels [15]. Enhanced depth imaging optical coherence tomography (EDI-OCT) shows increased subfoveal choroidal thickness even in eyes without evident uveitis activity, making this finding a possible indicator of subclinical ocular inflammation in patients with BD [16].

Optic neuropathy (ON), although considered a rare manifestation of Behcet´s disease, might actually be overshadowed by uveitis' complications. It can appear during the course of already known BD (and should be considered as part of the neuro-BD disease spectrum), or it can even be the first manifestation of the disease (BD should then be kept in mind as a differential diagnosis of optic neuropathy

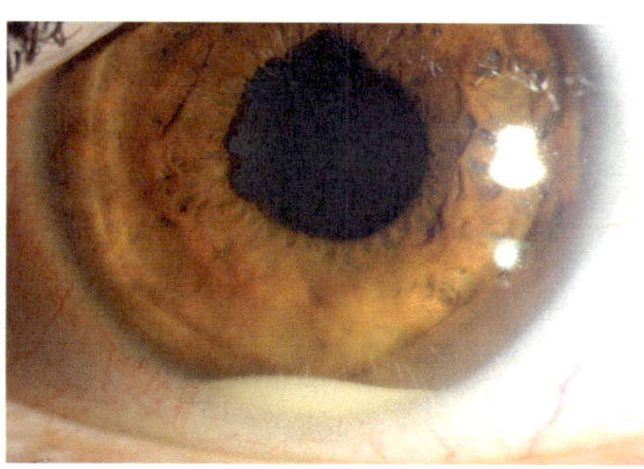

**Figure 1.**
*Hypopyon and nasal synechiae in the left eye of a young patient suffering from acute reactivation of anterior uveitis related to Behcet's disease.*

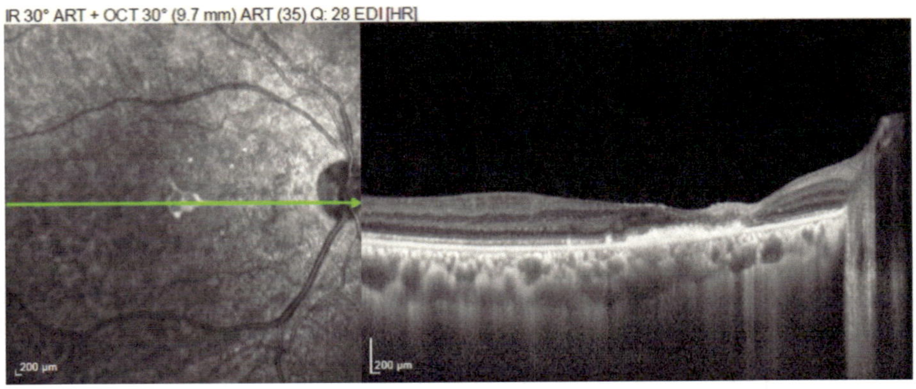


**Figure 2.**
*Horizontal OCT scan from the right eye of a patient with advanced Behcet's disease posterior uveitis. Generalized retinal atrophy and retinal pigment hypertrophy are seen.*

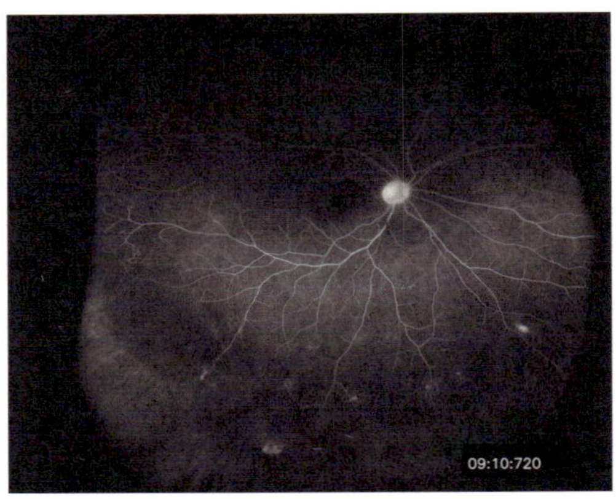


**Figure 3.**
*Late-frame fluorescein angiography showing extensive peripheral areas of retinal non-perfusion affecting the inferior temporal area of the right eye.*

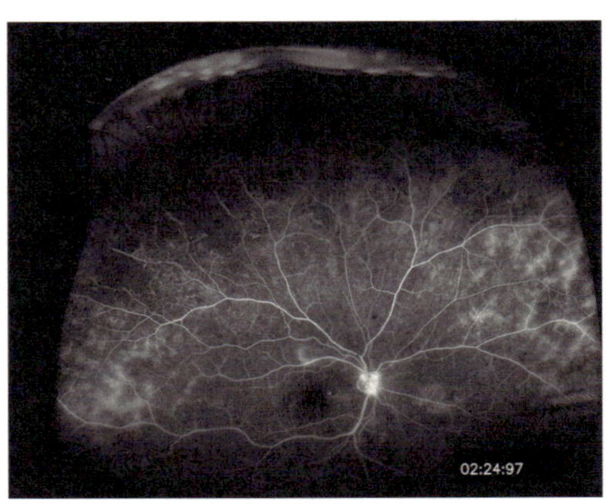


**Figure 4.**
*Early frame fluorescein angiography of the right eye of a patient suffering from Behcet's disease retinal vasculitis. Areas of capillary leakage are present as well as peripheral ischemia and optic disc hyperfluorescence.*

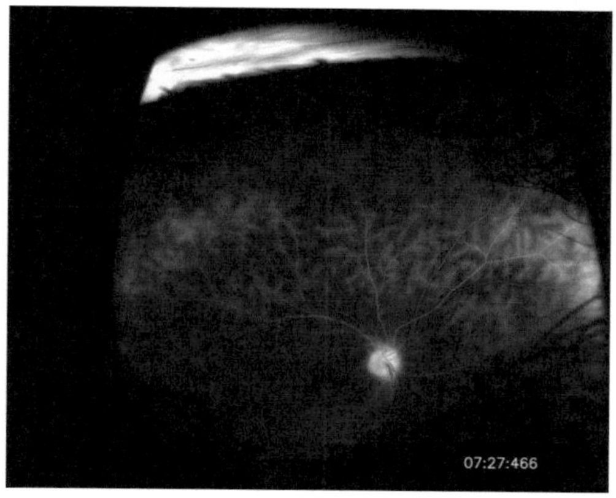


**Figure 5.**
*Late-frame fluorescein angiography of the right and left eye from a patient suffering from Behcet's disease associated with retinal vasculitis. Typical "fern-leaf" pattern of capillary leakage is present.*

in regions where its prevalence is high) [17]. The prognosis of BD-associated ON seems not to be as poor as the one of BD uveitis, with excellent response to the combination of corticosteroids and immunosuppressants and recovery as the rule [18, 19]. However, the use of cyclosporine should be avoided in these cases since it could promote the development of neurologic involvement [20].

## 3. Etiology and pathogenesis

Despite years of research, BD remains idiopathic. Even though there are sporadic cases all around the world, disease is more prevalent along the ancient silk route and in countries located between 30 and 45 north latitude through the Mediterranean Basin, the Middle East, and Far East regions such as China and Japan [21]. This particular geographic distribution points toward a genetic predisposing factor. The high frequency of HLA-B51 among a wide range of affected ethnic populations highlights the importance of a special genetic background: even though not considered as part of the diagnostic criteria, the positivity of HLA-B51 increases the risk of BD in around six times [22].

Besides the classic and well-known predisposition to BD associated with HLA-B51 positivity, new insights on disease's pathogenesis came out from genome-wide association studies (GWAS). The disruption of different biological pathways might determine the intrinsic biological process in multifactorial diseases, as BD. Six biologic pathways have been recently identified as possible mechanisms in the pathogenesis of BD:focal adhesion pathway, MAPK (mitogen-activated protein kinase) signaling, TGF (transforming growth factor) beta signaling, ECM-receptor interaction, complement and coagulation cascades and proteasome pathways [23].

Then, on this special genetic background, environmental factors might play a role as triggers for disease development. Infectious agents have been postulated as these triggering factors. Recently, a relationship between periodontal disease and specific polymorphisms of interleukin (IL)-1alpha and (IL)-1beta in Turkish patients with BD was reported, making periodontitis-induced autoinflammatory response a candidate for the development or severity of BD via IL-1 gene alteration [24]. Improvement of oral health among this high-risk population might affect BD course, leading to a better prognosis [25].

Neutrophils' activation plays a predominant role in BD; this is evidenced through the positivity of pathergy test, one of the diagnostic criteria for the disease [2, 26]. The activation of the innate immune system against environmental and/or autoantigens in this particular genetic background is then perpetuated by the adaptive immune system [27].

## 4. Diagnosis and differential diagnosis

As it was already stated, diagnosis is clinical and based on the presence of different combinations of symptoms and signs. In the acute attack, patients usually show raised inflammatory acute reactants (sedimentation rate and C-reactive protein) and high levels of white blood cells, mainly neutrophils [28, 29].

HLA-B51 is positive in around 50–70% of cases even though not necessary for the diagnosis [22, 30].

Differential diagnosis of hypopyon uveitis encompasses HLA-B27 associated, endogenous/exogenous endophthalmitis, toxic anterior segment syndrome (TASS) after cataract surgery, and masquerade syndromes [31–35]. BD-associated retinal vasculitis is unique in its predilection for capillaries but a similar picture can eventually be found in cases of HLA-B27 posterior uveitis with retinal vasculitis [36–39].

## 5. Treatment

Topical treatment is reserved for the minority of cases in which anterior uveitis is the only ocular disease manifestation. Prednisolone acetate with or without cyclopentolate is usually enough to stop episodes of anterior non-granulomatous uveitis. However, if these attacks are frequent or inflammatory quiescence requires more than three drops per day of prednisolone acetate for long periods, systemic treatment should be initiated.

The majority of cases presenting with posterior uveitis will require systemic treatment to control the sight-threatening manifestations of the disease.

High-dose systemic corticosteroids (1 g intravenous of Solu-Medrol or 1 mg/kg/day of oral prednisone) are useful in severe acute inflammatory attacks. However, they should not be administered alone given the high risk of flare up while tapering and the side effect profile of high doses [40].

Azathioprine and cyclosporine have both shown to be effective in BD's uveitis in two different randomized clinical trials (RCT) [41–43]. In many cases, a single agent is not enough to control uveitis, and a combination of them is administered. Drugs are usually well tolerated in long term, providing the proper check of their own side effects' profile is performed (liver toxicity for azathioprine, renal toxicity for cyclosporine). The likelihood of patients on cyclosporine to develop CNS complications should be kept in mind, and the drug is not recommended in the management of BD's associated optic neuropathy [44].

High levels of tumor necrosis factor (TNF) alpha are present in BD's uveitis [45]. The blockage of this inflammatory pathway is therefore a very effective approach to disease control. Infliximab (a chimeric monoclonal antibody against TNF alpha) and adalimumab (a fully humanized monoclonal antibody) are both widely used in the treatment of BD-associated posterior uveitis with high rates of success [46]. Adalimumab has the advantage of subcutaneous administration, theoretically improving patients' quality of life [47].

Other anti-TNF alpha molecules, such as certolizumab pegol and golimumab, have also shown positive results in small case series of BD's uveitis [48, 49].

Interferon alpha-2a is a very effective biologic treatment for BD's associated posterior uveitis [50]. Subcutaneously administered, it has rapid positive effect and also long relapse-free period making prophylactic maintenance treatment unnecessary [51, 52]. Drug is administered as a monotherapy after discontinuation of all previous immunosuppressive drugs (including corticosteroids). However, the associated flu-like syndrome limits the use of this important agent in the management of BD's uveitis.

Cytotoxic agents (chlorambucil and cyclophosphamide) were in the past the drug of choice for this severe form of uveitis [53, 54]. Nowadays, however, given the more specific and less toxic agents available, they are only used in those settings

Intravitreal steroids (either triamcinolone acetonide, fluocinolone, or dexamethasone implant) are adjuvant rescue treatment in recalcitrant cases not responding to systemic medication or whenever systemic medication is contraindicated [55]. Their effect is always transitory and associated with the risk of local complications (mainly cataract and glaucoma).

## 6. Prognosis

Visual prognosis is directly related to anatomical location of inflammation and rapid introduction of proper treatment. The minority of cases manifesting only by anterior uveitis usually shows excellent visual prognosis. Posterior uveitis, however, might be sight-threatening even if only one acute attack involves the macula. The development of modern biologic agents has positively changed the natural guarded prognosis of this disease even though there is still a low proportion of cases that will not respond to different combinations of treatment.

## Author details

Karina Julian[1,2]* and Bahram Bodaghi[3]

1 Eye Institute, Cleveland Clinic Abu Dhabi, Abu Dhabi, United Arab Emirates

2 Cleveland Clinic Lerner College of Medicine, Case Western Reserve University, United States

3 IHU FOReSIGHT, Sorbonne University, Pitié-Salpêtrière Hospital, Paris, France

*Address all correspondence to: karinajulian@hotmail.com

## References

[1] Behçet H. On relapsing, aphthous ulcers of the mouth, eye and genitalia caused by a virus. Clinical and Experimental Rheumatology. 2010. DOI: 10.1016/j.irle.2009.01.004

[2] International Study Group for Behçet's Disease. Criteria for diagnosis of Behcet's disease. Lancet. 1990. DOI: 10.1016/0140-6736(90)92643-V

[3] Davatchi F. Diagnosis/classification criteria for Behcet's disease. Pathology Research International. 2012. DOI: 10.1155/2012/607921

[4] Dilsen N. History and development of Behcet's disease. Revue du Rhumatisme (English Ed.). 1996

[5] Davatchi F, Sadeghi Abdollahi B, Chams-Davatchi C, et al. The saga of diagnostic/classification criteria in Behcet's disease. International Journal of Rheumatic Diseases. 2015. DOI: 10.1111/1756-185X.12520

[6] Kronborg C, Mahar PD, Kelly R. Should we keep changing the diagnostic criteria for Behçet's disease? Dermatology. 2014. DOI: 10.1159/000355481

[7] Scherrer MAR, Rocha VB, Garcia LC. Behçet´s disease: Review with emphasis on dermatological aspects. Anais Brasileiros de Dermatologia. 2017. DOI: 10.1590/abd1806-4841.20177359

[8] Fatemi A, Shahram F, Akhlaghi M, Smiley A, Nadji A, Davatchi F. Prospective study of articular manifestations in Behçet's disease: Five-year report. International Journal of Rheumatic Diseases. 2017. DOI: 10.1111/1756-185X.12633

[9] Zhu Z, Shu X, Long S, et al. Ulcerative colitis followed by the development of typical intestinal Behçet disease. Med (United States). 2018. DOI: 10.1097/MD.0000000000009882

[10] Akman-Demir G, Serdaroglu P, Tasçi B. Clinical patterns of neurological involvement in Behcet's disease: Evaluation of 200 patients. Brain. 1999. DOI: 10.1093/brain/122.11.2171

[11] Koc Y, Gullu I, Akpek G, et al. Vascular involvement in Behcet's disease. The Journal of Rheumatology. 1992. DOI: 10.1016/j.revmed.2009.09.024

[12] Zeghidi H, Saadoun D, Bodaghi B. Les manifestations oculaires de la maladie de Behçet. La Revue de Médecine Interne. 2014. DOI: 10.1016/j.revmed.2013.10.011

[13] Takeuchi M, Iwasaki T, Kezuka T, et al. Functional and morphological changes in the eyes of Behçet's patients with uveitis. Acta Ophthalmologica. 2010. DOI: 10.1111/j.1755-3768.2009.01536.x

[14] Tugal-Tutkun I, Ozdal PC, Oray M, Onal S. Review for diagnostics of the year: Multimodal imaging in Behçet uveitis. Ocular Immunology and Inflammation. 2017. DOI: 10.1080/09273948.2016.1205100

[15] Atmaca LS, Sonmez PA. Fluorescein and indocyanine green angiography findings in Behcet's disease. The British Journal of Ophthalmology. 2003. DOI: 10.1136/bjo.87.12.1466

[16] Chung Y-R, Cho EH, Jang S, Lee SY, Lee E-S, Lee K. Choroidal thickness indicates subclinical ocular and systemic inflammation in eyes with Behçet disease without active inflammation. Korean Journal of Ophthalmology. 2018. DOI: 10.3341/kjo.2017.0139

[17] Akdal G, Toydemir HE, Saatci AO, et al. Characteristics of optic neuropathy in Behçet disease. Neurology: Neuroimmunology & Neuroinflammation. 2018. DOI: 10.1212/NXI.0000000000000490

[18] Kidd DP. Optic neuropathy in Behçet's syndrome. Journal of Neurology. 2013. DOI: 10.1007/s00415-013-7070-4

[19] Khanfir MS, Belfeki N, Said F, et al. Inflammatory optic neuropathy in Behçet's disease. Reumatismo. 2015. DOI: 10.4081/jlimnol.2014.817

[20] Akmar-Demir G, Ayranci O, Kurtuncu M, Vanli EN, Mutlu M, Tugal-Tutkun I. Cyclosporine for Behçet's uveitis: Is it associated with an increased risk of neurological involvement? Clinical and Experimental Rheumatology. Jul-Aug 2008;**26**(4 Suppl 50):S84-S90

[21] Alpsoy E. Behçet's disease: A comprehensive review with a focus on epidemiology, etiology and clinical features, and management of mucocutaneous lesions. The Journal of Dermatology. 2016. DOI: 10.1111/1346-8138.13381

[22] De Menthon M, LaValley MP, Maldini C, Guillevin L, Mahr A. HLA-B51/B5 and the risk of Behçet's disease: A systematic review and meta-analysis of case-control genetic association studies. Arthritis Care and Research. 2009. DOI: 10.1002/art.24642

[23] Bakir-Gungor B, Remmers EF, Meguro A, et al. Identification of possible pathogenic pathways in Behçet's disease using genome-wide association study data from two different populations. European Journal of Human Genetics. 2015. DOI: 10.1038/ejhg.2014.158

[24] Akman A, Ekinci NC, Kacaroglu H, Yavuzer U, Alpsoy E, Yegin O. Relationship between periodontal findings and specific polymorphisms of interleukin-1α and -1β in Turkish patients with Behçet's disease. Archives of Dermatological Research. 2008. DOI: 10.1007/s00403-007-0794-1

[25] Mumcu G, Ergun T, Inanc N, et al. Oral health is impaired in Behçet's disease and is associated with disease severity. Rheumatology. 2004. DOI: 10.1093/rheumatology/keh236

[26] Davatchi F, Chams-Davatchi C, Ghodsi Z, et al. Diagnostic value of pathergy test in Behcet's disease according to the change of incidence over the time. Clinical Rheumatology. 2011. DOI: 10.1007/s10067-011-1694-5

[27] Direskeneli H. Autoimmunity vs autoinflammation in Behcet's disease: Do we oversimplify a complex disorder? Rheumatology. 2006. DOI: 10.1093/rheumatology/kel329

[28] Fordham JN, Davies PG, Kirk A, Currey HLF. Polymorphonuclear function in Behcet's syndrome. Annals of the Rheumatic Diseases. 1982. DOI: 10.1136/ard.41.4.421

[29] Garcia Garcia O, Vidaller Palacin A, Munoz Sanchez J, Roca Linares G. [Granulocyte-apheresis in ocular Behcet's disease resistant to medical treatment]. Archivos de la Sociedad Española de Oftalmología. Spanish; Jul 2004;79(7):335-340

[30] Wallace GR, Niemczyk E. Genetics in ocular inflammation-basic principles. Ocular Immunology and Inflammation. 2011. DOI: 10.3109/09273948.2010.543306

[31] Mamalis N, Edelhauser HF, Dawson DG, Chew J, LeBoyer RM, Werner L. Toxic anterior segment syndrome. Journal of Cataract and Refractive Surgery. 2006. DOI: 10.1016/j.jcrs.2006.01.065

[32] Zaidi AA, Ying GS, Daniel E, et al. Hypopyon in patients with uveitis. Ophthalmology. 2010. DOI: 10.1016/j.ophtha.2009.07.025

[33] Iannetti L, Corsi C, Iafrate F, Sammartino P, Di Giorgio A, Pezzi PP. Bilateral uveitis with hypopyon as a presenting symptom of metastatic peritoneal carcinomatosis. European Journal of Ophthalmology. 2010

[34] Sudharshan S, Kumari A, Biswas J. Bilateral hypopyon as the presenting feature of chronic myeloid leukemia. Ocular Immunology and Inflammation. 2008. DOI: 10.1080/09273940802411437

[35] Corriveau C, Easterbrook M, Payne D. Lymphoma simulating uveitis (masquerade syndrome). Canadian Journal of Ophthalmology. 1986

[36] Sharma R, Randhawa S. Hemorrhagic ischemic retinal vasculitis and alopecia areata as a manifestation of HLA-B27. Ophthalmic Surg Lasers Imaging Retina. 2018. DOI: 10.3928/23258160-20171215-10

[37] Pathanapitoon K, Dodds EM, Cunningham ET, Rothova A. Clinical spectrum of HLA-B27-associated ocular inflammation. Ocular Immunology and Inflammation. 2017. DOI: 10.1080/09273948.2016.1185527

[38] Braakenburg AM, Rothova A. The clinical characteristics of retinal vasculitis in HLA-B27-positive patients. Ocular Immunology and Inflammation. 2014. DOI: 10.3109/09273948.2013.835429

[39] Dodds EM, Lowder CY, Meisler DM. Posterior segment inflammation in HLA-B27+ acute anterior uveitis: Clinical characteristics. Ocular Immunology and Inflammation. 1999;7(2):85-92. DOI: 10.1076/ocii.7.2.85.4015

[40] Reed JB, Morse LS, Schwab IR. High-dose intravenous pulse methylprednisolone hemisuccinate in acute Behcet retinitis. American Journal of Ophthalmology. 1998. DOI: 10.1016/S0002-9394(99)80163-9

[41] Yazici H, Pazarli H, Barnes CG, et al. A controlled trial of azathioprine in Behçet's syndrome. The New England Journal of Medicine. 1990. DOI: 10.1056/NEJM199002013220501

[42] Saadoun D, Wechsler B, Terrada C, et al. Azathioprine in severe uveitis of Behçet's disease. Arthritis Care & Research (Hoboken). 2010. DOI: 10.1002/acr.20308

[43] Masuda K, Urayama A, Kogure M, Nakajima A, Nakae K, Inaba G. Double-masked trial of cyclosporin versus colchicine and long-term open study of cyclosporin in Behçet's disease. Lancet. 1989. DOI: 10.1016/S0140-6736(89)92381-7

[44] Kotake S, Higashi K, Yoshikawa K, Sasamoto Y, Okamoto T, Matsuda H. Central nervous system symptoms in patients with Behcet disease receiving cyclosporine therapy. Ophthalmology. 1999. DOI: 10.1016/S0161-6420(99)90120-3

[45] Nalbant S, Sahan B, Durna M, et al. Cytokine profile in Behçet uveitis. Bratislava Med J. 2008. DOI: 10.1016/j.solmat.2011.10.028

[46] Imrie FR, Dick AD. Biologics in the treatment of uveitis. Current Opinion in Ophthalmology. 2007. DOI: 10.1097/ICU.0b013e3282f03d42

[47] Ramanan AV, Benton D, Compeyrot-Lacassagne S, Dawoud D, Hardwick B, Hickey H, et al. A randomised controlled trial of the clinical effectiveness, safety and cost-effectiveness of adalimumab in combination with methotrexate for the treatment of juvenile idiopathic arthritis associated uveitis (SYCAMORE Trial). Trials. 2014. DOI: 10.1109/ICM.2008.5393823

[48] Lopalco G, Emmi G, Gentileschi S, et al. Certolizumab Pegol treatment in Behcet's disease with different organ involvement: A multicenter retrospective observational study. Modern Rheumatology. 2017. DOI: 10.1080/14397595.2017.1285857

[49] Vitale A, Emmi G, Lopalco G, et al. Long-term efficacy and safety of golimumab in the treatment of

multirefractory Behçet's disease. Clinical Rheumatology. 2017. DOI: 10.1007/s10067-017-3627-4

[50] Yalçindağ FN, Uzun A. Results of interferon alpha-2a therapy in patients with Behcet's disease. Journal of Ocular Pharmacology and Therapeutics. 2012. DOI: 10.1089/jop.2011.0238

[51] Diwo E, Gueudry J, Saadoun D, Weschler B, LeHoang P, Bodaghi B. Long-term efficacy of interferon in severe uveitis associated with Behçet disease. Ocular Immunology and Inflammation. 2017. DOI: 10.1080/09273948.2016.1206204

[52] Onal S, Kazokoglu H, Koc A, et al. Long-term efficacy and safety of low-dose and dose-escalating interferon alfa-2a therapy in refractory Behçet uveitis. Archives of Ophthalmology. 2011. DOI: 10.1001/archophthalmol.2011.3

[53] Mudun BA, Ergen A, Ipcioglu SU, Burumcek EY, Durlu Y, Arslan MO. Short-term chlorambucil for refractory uveitis in Behcet's disease. Ocular Immunology and Inflammation. 2001. DOI: 10.1007/s00066-005-1394-7

[54] Davatchi F, Sadeghi Abdollahi B, Shams H, et al. Combination of pulse cyclophosphamide and azathioprine in ocular manifestations of Behcet's disease: Longitudinal study of up to 10 years. International Journal of Rheumatic Diseases. 2014. DOI: 10.1111/1756-185X.12248

[55] Fabiani C, Emmi G, Lopalco G, et al. Intravitreal dexamethasone implant as an adjunct weapon for severe and refractory uveitis in Behçet's disease. The Israel Medical Association Journal. 2017

Section 2

# Infectious Uveitis

Chapter 4

# Viral Retinitis: Diagnosis and Management Update

*Abhinav Dhami and Ravinder Kaur Malhi*


## Abstract

Cytomegalovirus, herpes simplex, and herpes zoster are responsible for the majority of cases of viral retinitis and can occur in both healthy and immunocompromised or immunodeficient individuals. Herpes zoster has been strongly incriminated as a causal agent in acute retinal necrosis in immunocompetent patients. Epstein Barr virus has been described in various ocular inflammatory diseases including multifocal choroiditis in healthy patients. In immunocompromised or immunodeficient patients, various opportunistic viral infections can occur; the most common being cytomegalovirus (CMV) infection. Other less common viruses causing retinal infections include herpes simplex virus (HSV) and varicella zoster virus (VZV). The vision-threatening complications associated with infectious viral disease are disastrous in nature due to rapid progression. The inability to control this viral retinitis requires early detection by the clinician with prompt and aggressive initiation of the drug therapy to prevent complications.


**Keywords:** acute retinal necrosis, herpes zoster, herpes simplex, cytomegalovirus

## 1. Introduction

Viral retinitis is an important vision threatening infectious disease of the retina which can occur in both immunocompetent and immunocompromised or immunodeficient acquired immunodeficiency syndrome (AIDS) individuals. In immunocompetent patients, acute retinal necrosis (ARN) has been recognized as a vision threatening inflammation caused primarily by herpes group of viruses while Epstein Barr virus (EBV) is associated with various ocular inflammatory diseases including multifocal choroiditis in healthy patients [1]. The immunocompromised or immunodeficient patients are predisposed to a higher risk for viral infections with the most common being cytomegalovirus (CMV) infection and the less commonly affecting viruses include herpes simplex virus (HSV) and varicella zoster virus (VZV) [1].

## 2. Acute retinal necrosis

It is characterized by the initial onset of episcleritis or scleritis, periorbital pain, and anterior uveitis, which may be granulomatous or stellate in appearance and lead to decreased vision resulting from vitreous opacification (**Figure 1a**), necrotizing retinitis, and, in some cases, optic neuritis or neuropathy. The American Uveitis Society released its criteria for diagnosis of acute retinal necrosis syndrome in 1994 (**Table 1**) [2]. Takase et al. [3] described a newer diagnostic criteria which includes: six ocular findings in the early stage, five clinical courses, and the virologic tests of intraocular fluids.

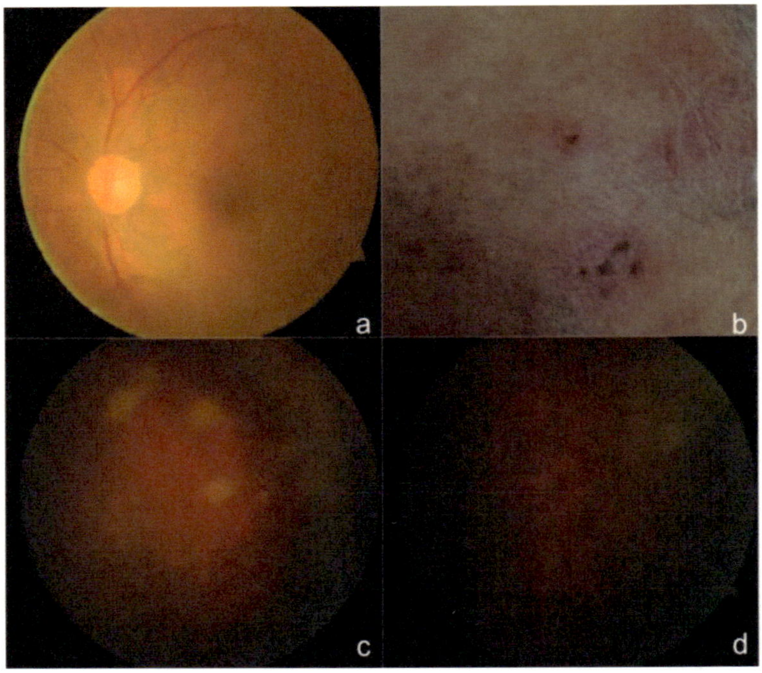


**Figure 1.**
*(a) Fundus photo of left eye showing media haze with vitritis, (b) herpes zoster lesions on the scalp, (c) peripheral fundus pictures showing deep yellowish white patches, in the peripheral retina and spreading concentrically with adjoining active vasculitis, and (d) resolution of the whitish lesion with valacyclovir 1 g TDS after 6 weeks.*

| Required clinical criteria | Supporting clinical criteria |
|---|---|
| One or more foci of retinal necrosis with discrete borders, located in peripheral retina | Optic neuropathy/atrophy |
| Rapid progression of disease in the absence of therapy | Scleritis |
| Circumferential spread of disease | Pain |
| Evidence of occlusive vasculopathy and arteriolar involvement | |
| A prominent inflammatory reaction in the vitreous and anterior chamber | |

**Table 1.**
*American uveitis society criteria for diagnosis of acute retinal necrosis.*

## 2.1 The six ocular findings include

(1a) Presence of anterior chamber cells or mutton-fat keratic precipitates.

(1b) Presence of yellow-white lesion in the peripheral retina (granular or patchy in the early stage, then gradually merging.

(1c) Associated retinal arteritis.

(1d) Presence of hyperemic optic disc.

(1e) Presence of inflammatory vitreous opacities.

(1f) Associated elevated intraocular pressure (IOP).

### 2.2 The five clinical courses include

(2a) Rapid expansion of retinal lesion circumferentially.

(2b) Development of retinal breaks or retinal detachment.

(2c) Associated retinal vascular occlusion.

(2d) Associated optic atrophy.

(2e) Response to antiviral agents.

### 2.3 Virologic testing

It consists of the intraocular fluid analysis by using PCR or the Goldmann-Witmer (GW) coefficient for HSV-1, HSV-2, or VZV. A "virus-confirmed ARN" was defined as the presence of ocular findings in stage 1a and 1b, the presence of any one of the five clinical courses, and a positive virologic test result. A "virus-unconfirmed ARN" was defined by them as the presence of four of six early stage ocular findings including 1a and 1b, presence of any two of the five clinical courses, a negative virologic test result, or when virologic testing had not been performed [3].

Clinical appearance of retinitis is deep yellowish white patches, typically beginning in the peripheral retina and spreading concentrically and towards the posterior pole (**Figure 1c** and **d**). An active vasculitis (**Figure 1a**) is present, with perivascular hemorrhages, sheathing, and terminal obliteration of arterioles by thrombi lasting about 4–6 weeks [4, 5].

Frequently the necrotic and normal retinal edge acts a site for developing fresh retinal breaks, with a 75% risk for developing rhegmatogenous retinal detachment (RRD) in untreated eyes [6]. Systemically these patients have a risk for developing meningoencephalitis and a neurologic symptoms should be borne in mid while treating such patients [7, 8].

## 3. Etiology

Considerable evidence points to multiple members of the herpesvirus family in the etiology of ARN syndrome with VZV (**Figure 1b**) [7] being the leading cause followed HSV [9] and rarely by CMV and EBV [10].

### 3.1 Histopathology

Studies of blind eyes enucleated early in the course of ARN have demonstrated retinal necrosis with eosinophilic intranuclear inclusions within cells of all layers of retina and retinal pigment epithelium. Immune complex deposition for VZV and HSV antigen can be noted in the retinal vessels [11].

The differential diagnosis that need to be rules out include CMV retinopathy, syphilitic retinitis, toxoplasmosis, large cell lymphoma, hemorrhagic vasculitis and Progressive outer retinal necrosis [10].

ARN is a syndrome whose clinical diagnosis is established on the basis of the evolving signs and symptoms, which may be pathognomonic in many cases, but in atypical cases ancillary clinical history or laboratory tests help in supporting and identifying the diagnosis [1, 2]. The patient's level of immunocompetence has to be determined, as this adds knowledge of the seropositivity to HIV and syphilis and may help to establish an appropriate and specific diagnosis. The most sensitive and specific method for the detection of herpes viruses in vitreous specimens is the polymerase chain reaction (PCR) [3–7]. Genomic DNA of human herpes virus (HHV), toxoplasma, bacteria, and fungi can be measured in the aqueous humor and vitreous fluids using of two independent PCR assays either a qualitative multiplex PCR or a quantitative real-time PCR and secondly a broad-range real-time PCR. The multiplex PCR can qualitatively measures the genomic DNA of eight different types of HHVs: (HSV) type 1 (HHV-1), HSV-2 (HHV-2), (VZV; HHV-3), Epstein-Barr virus (EBV; HHV-4), CMV (HHV-5), HHV-6, HHV-7, HHV-8, and toxoplasma [3]. PCR is now capable of detecting a single varicella zoster with a positivity of 86.4% and it was noted that aqueous sample yields a lesser chance for detection of virion in comparison to vitreous biopsy [12, 13].

Takase et al. [3] observed the overall rate of positive results of PCR for HSV-1, HSV-2, or VZV was 95% for ARN and 8% for control uveitis, a difference that was statistically significant [3]. In cases in which PCR is negative but a high clinical suspicion, endoretinal biopsy and a central spinal fluid tap has been deemed more appropriate. Taking the biopsy from the transition zone between normal and necrotic retina during the acute phase of the disease greatly increases its diagnostic yield [12]. Another method for detection of intraocular viral infection can be achieved by measuring the viral antibody titers (FA) in serum and intraocular fluids and then calculating the quotient ratio (Q value or Goldmann-Witmer coefficient). If the Goldmann-Witmer coefficient of 1 or above is obtained, it is establishes proof of intraocular specific antibody production, hence intraocular infection should be suspected. However, the positivity of the Goldmann-Witmer coefficient can vary with time and from onset of ARN syndrome [3, 14].

## 4. Prognosis and treatment

Literature states that a generally poor prognosis in untreated eyes is expected in eyes with classic ARN syndrome and only 28% of affected eyes end up obtaining a final vision better than 20/200 as there are coexistent risks of RRD (75% of affected eyes), optic nerve dysfunction, or macular abnormality [6].

In the recent era of antiviral therapy and vitrectomy techniques have enabled in decreasing the level of vision loss associated with ARN to less than one-third of cases in recent years [15]. However, the use of prophylactic laser photocoagulation has become more controversial than it was in the past [16]. The comparison of lasered and non-lasered eyes as analyzed by Roy et al. [17], concluded that many eyes with severe ARN with the presence of vitreous inflammatory opacification usually preclude the application of laser, whereas eyes with mild ARN with relatively clear media allows the application of laser. They noted that prophylactic laser retinopexy failed to prevent secondary RD and found no protective role in preventing RRD's even after laser retinopexy, because the involved retinal area continues to extend posteriorly beyond the demarcation of the laser burns. It was concluded that eyes in which laser treatment was possible, obviously had less retinitis and hence vitritis, which ultimately gave them a better final visual prognosis [17].

## 5. Treatment

(1g) Acyclovir is given intravenously for 5–10 days of 1500 mg/m$^2$/day in three divided does with normal renal function tests. This is followed by oral acyclovir dose 800 mg (orally) 5 times daily for 6 weeks. The side-effects which close monitoring include decreased renal function, gastrointestinal irritation, phlebitis, central nervous system dysfunction, and hypersensitivity reactions. The most potent antiviral action is against VZV, HSV types 1 and 2, EBV, but a low activity has been noted in various studies against CMV [17].

(1h) Valacyclovir [L-valyl ester of acyclovir], has better bioavailability and is used in the doses of 1 g three times a day for 6–8 weeks. Treatment algorithms as cited in literature used oral valacyclovir 1 g 3 times daily, oral famciclovir 500 mg 3 times daily, or valganciclovir 450–900 mg 2 times daily until complete resolution of retinitis was observed [17, 18]. Renal function need to be monitored for all antivirals are administered on a long-term basis, especially in extremes of age.

(1i) Adjunctive role for intravitreal antiviral medication in the treatment of ARN syndrome has been explored in early remission of the retinitis. The original dose of ganciclovir used was 200 or 400 mcg in 0.1 ml, but nowadays the dose is 2 mg in 0.05–0.1 ml. The injections are given on a weekly basis. Intravitreal foscarnet in humans at a dose of 2.4 mg in 0.1 ml has also been reported to be safe and effective in treating retinitis caused by cytomegalovirus followed with a maintenance dose once a week, with a close monitoring for optic and retinal toxicity. Intravitreal therapy forms a part of palliation therapy for patients who are unable to tolerate or refuse systemic treatment, or as an adjunct in severe disease. However, studies have demonstrated efficacy as good as or better than intravenous treatment [18, 19].

(1j) Systemic corticosteroids also may limit intraocular inflammation and the vitreous reaction, but are generally begun only after 24–48 h of intravenous acyclovir/oral valacyclovir [20].

(1k) The combination of systemic and intravitreal therapy has been reported as new a treatment paradigm for patients with ARN. Flaxel et al. conducted a comparative case series and analyzed in 24 patients with ARN treated over a 20-year period. They had 12 patients in the study who received combination systemic and intravitreal antiviral therapy while 12 patients received only systemic therapy alone. Patients receiving combination therapy showed a higher incidence of two-line-or-greater visual acuity and decreased incidence of RD and severe visual acuity loss to 20/200 or poorer when compared to patients who received systemic antiviral alone and similar results were obtained by Wong et al. and Megphara et al. They concluded that patients that with moderate disease (i.e., 25–50% retina involved) usually showed better results. However, Tibbetts et al. found no statistically significant difference in the visual acuity and prevalence of retinal detachment with combination therapy [21].

In recent years the use of adjunctive intravitreal antivirals has increased as it enables a high concentration of antiviral agent to reach where it is needed most. Intravitreal foscarnet was used in 46.7% of patients by TF Cochrane et al. in their study and linked its use with a no specific reduction in the rate of retinal detachment versus eyes treated without intravitreal therapy. No specific guidelines have been outlined with the use and number of injections required for controlling the viral retinitis [13, 17, 18].

Kawaguchi et al. described an algorithm where they used combination of antiviral, anti-inflammatory and antithrombotic treatment depending on virus isolated. They suggested that higher doses of systemic acyclovir (10 vs. 15 mg/kg), oral prednisolone (30 vs. 40–60 mg/d) and aspirin (100 vs. 200–300 mg/d) should be given to those with VZV ARN [13]. Till date no specific trial has validated the efficacy of virus specific.

Treatment and all current treatment options available for ARN are based on anecdotal evidence.

Before the antiviral management the reported incidence of second eye involvement was 36% in ARN patients, usually within 6 weeks. However with better management, most of the recent studies conclude a fellow-eye involvement rate of around 3% with appropriate antiviral treatment [6, 18]. The duration for which the systemic treatment should be continued to prevent fellow-eye involvement is not well established in literature. The risk is believed to be decrease if therapy is continued for 6–12 weeks. The incidence of bilateral ARN reported in literature has been as late as 34 years after the first eye became affected [18]. The syndrome of ARN is a potentially visually devastating disorder with multifactorial pathogenesis. Its successful management depends on further advances in antiviral chemotherapy, control of the ischemic vasculopathy, and prevention of proliferative vitreoretinopathy [1, 5, 22].

To conclude ARN is a rare but potentially visually devastating condition and both qualitative and quantitative real-time PCR testing may be used both to ascertain the etiology of ARN and to assess the response to therapy. During the last few years the first-line of therapy has been the use of oral prodrugs valacyclovir, famciclovir and valganciclovir which has gained popularity because the patients do not have to be hospitalized with oral therapy in contrast to intravenous therapy and thus preventing the devastating complications. It is still a matter of debate from most of the studies whether and where all prophylactic laser is deemed beneficial in preventing RRD. Intravitreal antiviral therapy acts in supportive role in combination with the oral antiviral therapy for better visual outcomes.

## 6. Cytomegalovirus retinitis

CMV is ubiquitous entity and its seroprevalence rises from nearly 60% in patients 6 years or older to greater than 90% in individuals more than 80 year of age [23].

In immunocompetent individuals the initial infection with CMV causes minimal symptoms, although an associated mononucleosis-like syndrome can be a presentation. Cell-mediated immunity helps to control the virus and prevents specific organ disease in all, but may affect a few patients [24]. However, in the presence of advanced immunosuppression, such as AIDS, history of organ transplantation with iatrogenic immunosuppression, autoimmune disease, or malignancy are a higher risk of developing specific end-organ CMV disease (e.g., encephalitis, esophagitis, colitis, and retinitis), thus increasing the risk of morbidity and mortality [23–25].

## 7. Ophthalmoscopic findings

The diagnosis of CMV is based on clinical appearance and correlating it with a supportive history of an immunocompromised state. The retinal lesions appear peripherally in a perivascular distribution as a creamy white infiltrate and associated

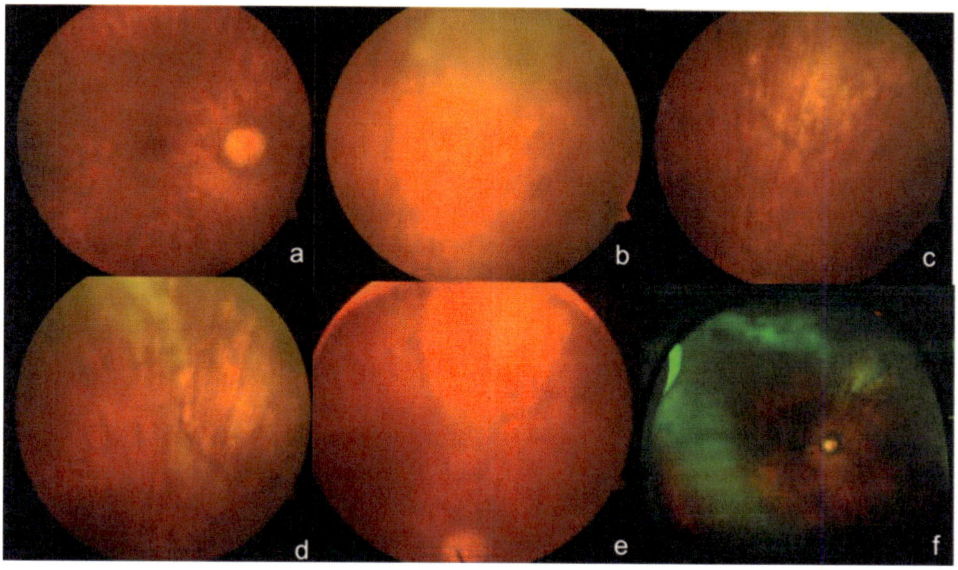


**Figure 2.**
*(a) Fundus picture of right eye of a female patient presented with diminution of vision after renal transplant, with posterior active vasculitis with presence of hemorrhages, (b) (superior retina just above the arcade) a mid-peripheral perivascular vitritis with a creamy white infiltrate, with a more granular border, (c) the area of resolution of the whitish lesion after treatment with 450 mg B.D of valganciclovir after 3 months, (d) recurrence at the edge of the lesion 2 months post tapering dose of valganciclovir, (e) resolution of the recurrence at the edge with initiation of 450 mg B.D of valganciclovir, and (f) an wide field image at last follow where patient underwent intravitreal ganciclovir injection 2 mg/0.5 ml with oral valganciclovir, showing resolution of the retinitis with peripheral scarring and gliosis.*

granular borders surrounded with smaller satellite lesions (**Figure 2a** and **b**). There is a space of "clear" retina separating in between the granular foci. Progression of active retinitis causes scarring (**Figure 2c**), suggesting the virus involvement from the beginning. The active border progresses posteriorly, at a rate of 250–350 μm/week, causing scarring and adjoining necrosis of retina (**Figure 2f**) with mottled pigmentation of the RPE. The term "pizza pie" appearance is associated with CMV if the retinitis lesions are presenting more posteriorly thus involving the retinal vessels and causing retinal hemorrhages (**Figure 2a**) [25, 26].

A second pattern of CMV retinitis has as describes includes a "granular" or "brushfire border." The focal granular infiltrates enlarge slowly and advancement is associated with destruction of the retina and leaving a atrophic retinal pigment epithelium behind. Hemorrhages and vitreous cells are less prominent seen. This is attributed to be direct cell-to cell transfer of infected virions in this pattern of infection. The brushfire border is commonly seen in the anterior to the equator [24–27].

The clinical appearance of newly diagnosed CMV retinitis has not altered appreciably from the pre-highly antiretroviral therapy (HAART) era to the HAART era [26]. A delay in diagnosis increases the risk of vision loss either due to fulminant retinitis (foveal or optic nerve involvement), or it may induce immune recovery uveitis (IRU) and its associated sequelae increase with the severity of CMV retinitis in elderly, healthy patients with CMV retinitis. The delayed diagnosis causes retinal arteriolar occlusions, with poor visual outcomes [27].

Histopathologically there is presence of extensive areas of necrosis with diffuse or full thickness retinal involvement. In the areas of necrosis intracytoplasmic as well intranuclear inclusions resembling 'Owl eyes' can be noted. The majority of the enlarged cells are in the range of 20–30 μm with intranuclear basophilic inclusion and numerous eosinophilic intracytoplasmic inclusions [28].

## 8. Clinical findings of CMV retinitis in non-HIV-positive patients

In elderly immune-competent patients (other than the natural waning of immunity and increased prevalence of typical comorbidities that come with age), CMV retinitis tends to have an increased association with retinal arteriolar occlusions, even with minimal retinitis. In patients with limited immune dysfunction (due to old age, diabetes, or noncytotoxic immunosuppression), CMV retinitis can present with typical peripheral, granular, and slowly progressive retinitis and an atypical panretinal occlusive vasculitis, mimicking ARN [29].

### 8.1 Biochemical testing

In cases of diagnostic dilemma, especially in the absence of an identifiable source of host immunosuppression, polymerase chain reaction (PCR) of aqueous or vitreous samples can amplify CMV DNA and secure a diagnosis. Recently, a loop-mediated isothermal amplification (LAMP) assay has demonstrated 100% concordance with PCR in detecting CMV DNA in vitreous samples of patients suspected or diagnosed as CMV retinitis at a fraction of the cost, potentially increasing the diagnostic capabilities of clinicians in [30, 31].

### 8.2 Screening

All HIV individuals with CD4+ T cell counts <50 cells/μL, need a screening by a uveitis or retinal specialist using dilated fundus exams every 3 months [27].

In patients undergoing allogenic hematopoietic stem cell transplantation (HSCT) after conditioning with an alemtuzumab (Campath, Genzyme, Cambridge, MA)-based regimen, the frequency of CMV retinitis can approach 24% and similarly, post-HSCT patients with a significant CMV viral load (peak CMV DNA level $>7.64 \times 10^4$ copies/mL) are at increased risk of developing CMV retinitis and require periodic screening for ruling out retinitis [32].

### 8.3 Management

Because no currently available agent is virucidal, the goal of therapy is to arrest viral replication/assembly until the host's immune system has recovered sufficiently to assume this function. Factors to be considered in selecting the mode of therapy include the patient's potential for immunologic improvement, the location and severity of CMV retinitis, and the risks, costs, and convenience associated with various therapies [32].

In the setting of HIV/AIDS, initiation of HAART is the most critical step in planning for long-term suppression of CMV retinitis. In the event that immune system recovery is unexpected (i.e., transplant recipients requiring lifelong immunosuppression), the physician should provide indefinite virostatic treatment [32].

The treatment for CMV retinitis includes three intravenous drugs: oral or intravenous ganciclovir, intravenous foscarnet and intravenous cidofovir. The role of systemic therapy is by starting at a higher induction dose for 2–3 weeks, followed by lower maintenance doses as it helps in preventing relapses of the retinitis. The purposed mechanism of action is specific selective inhibition of viral DNA polymerase [32].

The treatment of choice includes intravenous ganciclovir in in two divided doses for 2 weeks of initial induction therapy (5–7 mg/kg/day), followed by a once-daily maintenance dose. It is continued until the lesions begin to resolve and the patient's immune status shows improvement. Oral valganciclovir 900 mg twice daily as induction therapy followed by 900 mg once daily as maintenance dose as it serves an additional advantage of being a non-parenteral mode of treatment and avoiding complications relating to indwelling catheters, especially in immunocompromised patients. Foscarnet is administered as 90 mg/kg, twice daily for 14–21 days, as induction therapy, followed by once-daily administration as maintenance therapy. It is the preferred treatment of choice in Ganciclovir resistant cases [19, 32–34].

Recently the use of oral valganciclovir (Valcyte, Roche), an L-valyl ester prodrug of ganciclovir, is preferred as it obviates the risks due to intravenous therapy, but the cost of therapy and its related myelosuppression remain an issue. The bioavailability of 60% is obtained by the drug, which is comparable to intravenous ganciclovir and far greater than with oral ganciclovir (5%). Several newer antiviral agents are in various stages of preclinical experiments to phase 2 clinical trials include: Cidofovir, Maribavir (GlaxoSmithKline, Philadelphia, PA), BAY 38-4766 (Bayer, Pittsburgh, PA), and AIC246 (AiCuris, Wuppertal, Germany), inhibit viral activity through pathways other than the inhibition of viral DNA polymerase [33].

### 8.4 Intravitreal therapy

The preferred intravitreal injections consist of either ganciclovir or foscarnet, with or without systemic medication, to control sight-threatening retinitis. Induction dosing with intravitreal medications requires injections two to three times weekly, while once weekly generally is sufficient for maintenance.

1. Ganciclovir: the original dose used was 200 or 400 mcg in 0.1 ml, but almost all injections given today are 2 mg in 0.05–0.1 ml. The injections are given on a weekly basis. It is also available as an intraocular ganciclovir implant (Vitrasert, Bausch + Lomb, Rochester, NY) and demonstrated superiority over intravenous ganciclovir in terms of median time to the progression of retinitis (221 days for the 1 μg/h implant vs. 71 days for intravenous ganciclovir). Complication rates associated with the ganciclovir implant, most commonly for cataract, vitreous hemorrhage, and retinal detachment [20].

2. Foscarnet: it is used in the dose of 2.4 mg per 0.1 ml. It is used as twice weekly injections for induction period and once a week for maintenance therapy. They may be more effective in cases of resistant CMV disease. Combinations of high-dose intravitreal ganciclovir (3.0 mg twice a week) and foscarnet (2.4 mg twice a week) may be effective in patients who fail to respond or are intolerant to conventional therapy for ARN and HSV-1 retinitis. The most commonly reported complications include cataract, vitreous hemorrhage, and retinal detachment [34]

3. Cidofovir: the long half-life and potent anti-CMV activity of Cidofovir make it an attractive candidate for intravitreal injection. Studies in rabbits suggested that 100 mcg was a safe dose. Increased proteinuria and elevations in serum creatinine are the major dose limiting toxicities [19, 34, 35].

4. Fomivirsen: Vitravene, (Isis Pharmaceuticals Inc., Carlsbad, CA, USA) has also been studied for intravitreal use in patients with CMV retinitis, especially in situations where conventional therapy such as systemic and intravitreal ganciclovir, foscarnet, or cidofovir have failed or are contraindicated. Induction doses of fomivirsen are administered intravitreally at a dose of 330 mcg once every 2 weeks for 2 doses followed by maintenance therapy at same dose every 4 weeks [19, 34].

## 9. Treatment options in resistance

The treatment of CMV retinitis in the setting of drug resistance remains a particular challenge as newer antivirals take time to reach the level of commercial availability. Oral leflunomide (Arava, Sanofi-Aventis, Bridgewater, NJ), an immunosuppressive agent with anti-CMV activity, has demonstrated efficacy in transplant patients with systemic CMV infection and also in multi-drug-resistant CMV retinitis [36].

## 10. Conclusion

The evident benefits of HAART have helped in decreasing incidence and severity in immune compromised patients but still CMV retinitis remains the most common ocular opportunistic infection. Patients with a CD4+ T cell count <50 are at increased risk of CMV retinitis, and frequent screening of these patients is the need of the hour to detect the disease before it becomes sight-threatening [36].

### 10.1 Progressive outer retinal necrosis

Progressive outer retinal necrosis (PORN, also known as VZV retinitis or rapidly progressive herpetic retinal necrosis) was described and cited most by Engstrom and colleagues in 1994. They established about its devastating nature, in which two-thirds of eyes progressed to no light perception (NLP) within 4 weeks of onset. They concluded that most patients with this syndrome have had low CD4 cell counts (i.e., below 50/ml). It is mostly found in immunocompromised patients and diagnosis is based on the presence of:

1. Multifocal lesions with deep retinal opacification without granular borders with some areas of confluent opacification.

2. Peripheral retina location, with or without macular involvement.

3. Rapid progression.

4. Absence of vascular inflammation.

5. Minimal or no intraocular inflammation.

6. Perivascular clearing of the retinal opacification (hallmark of PORN syndrome).

7. Immunocompromised or patients with immunosuppression [37, 38].

Therapy of PORN often requires immediate high-dose anti-zoster or -HSV therapy. The earliest reports of treatment of PORN with single intravenous antivirals, primarily acyclovir, showed poor visual results. Recently the studies have shown an improvement in the visual outcomes with the combination use of intravenous and intravitreal antiviral treatment [38].

Scott et al. have reported that final vision of 20/80 or better in 5 of 11 eyes (45%) and only two of 11 eyes (18%) progressing to NLP vision. This was achieved utilizing a regimen of intravitreal ganciclovir and foscarnet plus IV foscarnet and IV ganciclovir or oral valganciclovir [39].

Gore et al. have the largest published series of patients with PORN treated with intravitreal ganciclovir antiviral therapy, found an improvement in final vision, with only 9 (13%) eyes losing perception of light. They observed that the retinas in patients receiving HAART when first evaluated were significantly less likely to detach and had a bimodal distribution to retinal detachment, the vast majority of retinas detaching within the first few weeks (i.e., during the active necrotic phase) and a few detaching many months later (i.e., during the inactive phase). The early group can be explained by full-thickness necrosis, leading to holes though both the inner and outer retina, as a prelude to RRD. For delayed RRD's they proposed that some retina's are associated with one or more sieve-like holes that can occasionally self-seal with the ensuing scarring process, allowing a functioning retinal pigment epithelium to pump the detachment flat [39].

Despite some patients being able to retain workable good vision, the overall functional outcomes remain alarming as a result of the catastrophic loss of vision PORN can lead to. The most encouraging results are achieved with improved visual outcomes when associated with early response to intravitreal ganciclovir injections. The best outcomes are limited to be seen in patients who begin intravitreal (and systemic) therapy within a few days of symptom onset, before macular involvement is apparent [39].

## Sources of support

Nil. No proprietary interest or conflict. No financial funding disclosure.

## Author details

Abhinav Dhami* and Ravinder Kaur Malhi
Vitreo-Retina Department, Dhami Eye Care Hospital, Punjab, India

*Address all correspondence to: drabhinavdhami@gmail.com

## References

[1] Biswas J, Madhavan HN, Gopal L, Badrinath SS. Clinical features and virologic studies in viral retinitis. Indian Journal of Ophthalmology. 1995;**43**:6368

[2] Holland GN. Standard diagnostic criteria for the acute retinal necrosis syndrome. Executive Committee of the American Uveitis Society. American Journal of Ophthalmology. 1994;**117**(5):663-667

[3] Takase H, Okada AA, Goto H, Mizuki N, Namba K, Ohguro N, et al. Development and validation of new diagnostic criteria for acute retinal necrosis. Japanese Journal of Ophthalmology. 2015;**59**(1):14-20

[4] Duker JS, Nielsen JC, Eagle RC Jr, et al. Rapidly progressive acute retinal necrosis secondary to herpes simplex virus, type 1. Ophthalmology. 1990;**97**(12):1638-1643

[5] Margolis T, Irvine AR, Hoyt WF, et al. Acute retinal necrosis syndrome presenting with papillitis and arcuate neuroretinitis. Ophthalmology. 1988;**95**(7):937-940

[6] Fox GM, Blumenkranz M. Giant retinal pigment epithelial tears in acute retinal necrosis. American Journal of Ophthalmology. 1993;**116**(3):302-306

[7] Cardine S, Chaze PA, Bourcier F, et al. Bilateral acute retinal necrosis syndrome associated with meningoencephalitis caused by herpes simplex virus 2. A case report. Journal Français d'Ophtalmologie. 2004;**27**(7):795-800

[8] Soushi S, Ozawa H, Matsuhashi M, et al. Demonstration of varicella-zoster virus antigens in the vitreous aspirates of patients with acute retinal necrosis syndrome. Ophthalmology. 1988;**95**(10):1394-1398

[9] Ludwig IH, Zegarra H, Zakov ZN. The acute retinal necrosis syndrome. Possible herpes simplex retinitis. Ophthalmology. 1984;**91**(12):1659-1664

[10] Kramer S, Brummer C, Zierhut M. Epstein-Barr virus associated acute retinal necrosis. The British Journal of Ophthalmology. 2001;**85**(1):114

[11] Culbertson WW, Blumenkranz MS, Haines H, et al. The acute retinal necrosis syndrome. Part 2: Histopathology and etiology. Ophthalmology. 1982;**89**(12):1317-1325

[12] Short GA, Margolis TP, Kuppermann BD, et al. A polymerase chain reaction-based assay for diagnosing varicella-zoster virus retinitis in patients with acquired immunodeficiency syndrome. American Journal of Ophthalmology. 1997;**123**(2):157-164

[13] Cochrane TF, Silvestri G, McDowell C, Foot B, McAvoy CE. Acute retinal necrosis in the United Kingdom: Results of a prospective surveillance study. Eye. 2012;**26**(3):370

[14] Usui Y, Goto H. Overview and diagnosis of acute retinal necrosis syndrome. Seminars in Ophthalmology. 2008;**23**(4):275-283

[15] Pepose JS, Flowers B, Stewart JA, et al. Herpesvirus antibody levels in the etiologic diagnosis of the acute retinal necrosis syndrome. American Journal of Ophthalmology. 1992;**113**(3):248-256

[16] Litoff D, Catalano RA. Herpes zoster optic neuritis in human immunodeficiency virus infection. Archives of Ophthalmology. 1990;**108**(6):782-783

[17] Roy R, Pal BP, Mathur G, Rao C, Das D, Biswas J. Acute retinal necrosis: Clinical features, management and outcomes–a 10 year consecutive case series. Ocular Immunology and Inflammation. 2014;**22**(3):170-174

[18] Tibbetts MD, Shah CP, Young LH, et al. Treatment of acute retinal necrosis. Ophthalmology. 2010;**117**(4):818-824

[19] Wong R, Pavesio CE, Laidlaw DA, Williamson TH, Graham EM, Stanford MR. Acute retinal necrosis: The effects of intravitreal foscarnet and virus type on outcome. Ophthalmology. 2010;**117**(3):556-560

[20] Teoh SC, Ou X, Lim TH. Intravitreal ganciclovir maintenance injection for cytomegalovirus retinitis: Efficacy of a low-volume, intermediate-dose regimen. Ophthalmology. 2012;**119**(3):588-595

[21] Shantha JG, Weissman HM, Debiec MR, Albini TA, Yeh S. Advances in the management of acute retinal necrosis. International Ophthalmology Clinics. 2015;**55**(3):1

[22] Hillenkamp J, N'lle B, Bruns C, et al. Acute retinal necrosis: Clinical features, early vitrectomy, and outcomes. Ophthalmology. 2009;**116**(10):1971-1975

[23] Staras SA, Dollard SC, Radford KW, et al. Seroprevalence of cytomegalovirus infection in the United States, 1988-1994. Clinical Infectious Diseases. 2006;**43**:1143-1151

[24] Gallant JE, Moore RD, Richman DD, et al. Incidence and natural history of cytomegalovirus disease in patients with advanced human immunodeficiency virus disease treated with zidovudine. The Zidovudine Epidemiology Study Group. The Journal of Infectious Diseases. 1992;**166**:1223-1227

[25] Holland GN, Sison RF, Jatulis DE, et al. Survival of patients with the acquired immune deficiency syndrome after development of cytomegalovirus retinopathy. UCLA CMV Retinopathy Study Group. Ophthalmology. 1990;**97**:204-211

[26] Jabs DA, Van Natta ML, Holbrook JT, et al. Longitudinal study of the ocular complications of AIDS: 2. Ocular examination results at enrollment. Ophthalmology. 2007;**114**:787-793

[27] Kempen JH, Min YI, Freeman WR, et al. Studies of Ocular Complications of AIDS Research Group. Risk of immune recovery uveitis in patients with AIDS and cytomegalovirus retinitis. Ophthalmology. 2006;**113**:684-694

[28] Chiotan C, Radu L, Serban R, Cornăcel C, Cioboata M, Anghel A. Cytomegalovirus retinitis in HIV/AIDS patients. Journal of Medicine and Life. 15 Jun 2014;**7**(2):237

[29] Schneider EW, Elner SG, van Kuijk FJ, et al. Chronic retinal necrosis: Cytomegalovirus necrotizing retinitis associated with panretinal vasculopathy in non-HIV patients. Retina. 2013;**33**:1791-1799

[30] Tran TH, Rozenberg F, Cassoux N, et al. Polymerase chain reaction analysis of aqueous humour samples in necrotizing retinitis. The British Journal of Ophthalmology. 2003;**87**:79-83

[31] Reddy AK, Balne PK, Reddy RK, et al. Development and evaluation of loop-mediated isothermal amplification assay for rapid and inexpensive detection of cytomegalovirus DNA in vitreous specimens from suspected cases of viral retinitis. Journal of Clinical Microbiology. 2010;**48**:2050-2052

[32] Song WK, Min YH, Kim YR, et al. Cytomegalovirus retinitis after

hematopoietic stem cell transplantation with alemtuzumab. Ophthalmology. 2008;**115**:1766-1770

[33] Studies of ocular complications of AIDS Research Group in collaboration with the AIDS Clinical Trials Group. Mortality in patients with the acquired immunodeficiency syndrome treated with either foscarnet or ganciclovir for CMV retinitis. The New England Journal of Medicine. 1992;**326**:213-220

[34] Vadlapudi AD, Vadlapatla RK, Mitra AK. Current and emerging antiviral for the treatment of cytomegalovirus (CMV) retinitis: An update on recent patents. Recent Patents on Anti-Infective Drug Discovery. 2012;7:8-18

[35] Rahhal FM, Arevalo JF, Munguia D, Taskintuna I, de la Paz EC, Azen SP, et al. Intravitreal cidofovir for the maintenance treatment of cytomegalovirus retinitis. Ophthalmology. 1996;**103**(7):1078-1083

[36] Thorne JE, Jabs DA, Kempen JH, et al. Incidence of and risk factors for visual acuity loss among patients with AIDS and cytomegalovirus retinitis in the era of highly active antiretroviral therapy. Ophthalmology. 2006;**113**:1432-1440

[37] Gore DM, Gore SK, Visser L. Progressive outer retinal necrosis: Outcomes in the intravitreal era. Archives of Ophthalmology. 2012;**130**(6):700-706

[38] Galindez OA, Sabates NR, Whitacre MM, Sabates FN. Rapidly progressive outer retinal necrosis caused by varicella zoster virus in a patient infected with human immunodeficiency virus. Clinical Infectious Diseases. 1996;**22**(1):149-151

[39] Scott IU, Luu KM, Davis JL. Intravitreal antivirals in the management of patients with acquired immunodeficiency syndrome with progressive outer retinal necrosis. Archives of Ophthalmology. 2002;**120**:1219-1222

Chapter 5

# Tuberculosis and Immunosuppressive Treatment in Uveitis Patients

*François Willermain, Laure Caspers, Weber Celia and Dorine Makhoul*

## Abstract

Uveitis is reported to be related to tuberculosis in 0.2–20% of cases. This large range reflects prevalence variations of tuberculosis around the globe as well as differences in diagnostic criteria. In addition, patients with noninfectious uveitis are frequently treated by immunomodulatory drugs and are thus at risk of TB reactivation. Search for tuberculosis infection is thus an important aspect in the work-up of patients with uveitis, even in low prevalence area. In the work up of such patients, the first question to ask is whether the patient has been infected by mycobacterium tuberculosis or not. The second question is to determine whether the uveitis is due or linked to this mycobacterial infection or not. Classical tuberculosis screening tools are used to answer the first question (TST, IGRA and chest X ray). The answer to the second question is much more challenging and will require the exclusion of other causes, to consider epidemiological data and clinical signs, polymerase chain reaction (PCR) on ocular fluids and therapeutically treatment trial. Disease prevalence will greatly influence all proposed tests and the final diagnosis. Tuberculosis prevalence in Western countries has progressively decreased during the twentieth century but remains elevated in cities with large migrating populations and drug addicts, with an increase of ultra-resistant cases. All those data must be carefully analyzed in order to collect enough evidences supporting tuberculosis uveitis before the initiation of a treatment with potential serious side and adapt the treatment to the increasing resistance.

**Keywords:** tuberculosis, uveitis, immunosuppressive agents, immunomodulatory agents

## 1. Introduction

Tuberculosis (TB) is a worldwide problem and a main concern for the World Health Organization. Nowadays, 30% of the human population is infected with the Koch bacillus and tuberculosis remains one of the major health problems on earth [1–4]. In 2014 alone, 9.6 million people were thought to be infected with Mycobacterium tuberculosis (Mtb) globally, in the vast majority of cases, infection leads to a latent form of tuberculosis, active disease being found in only 10% [1]. Latent tuberculosis (LTBI) occurs when individuals have been exposed to TB but remained systemically healthy. This latency relies on the presence of an active



IntechOpen

immune response against Mtb. All those people are thus at risk of TB reactivation in case of immunodepression. With area of globalization, all countries are affected with varying rates of infection, with high endemic countries from where migrant groups settle.

Uveitis is reported to be related to tuberculosis in 0.2–20% of cases [5]. This large range reflects prevalence variations of tuberculosis around the globe as well as differences in diagnostic criteria. The etiological relationship between tuberculosis and ocular inflammation is complex. Hence, direct demonstration of the presence of Mtb inside the eye is fairly rare because of the pauci-bacillary nature of the infection. If the patient has the evidence of systemic active TB infection, the uveitis may indicate direct ocular involvement by Mtb. However, in most cases, a diagnosis of presumed ocular tuberculosis will be made on the basis of the presence of compatible ophthalmological signs in the setting of a systemic (usually latent) infection [6–8]. In this context, recent studies suggest that in patients with vision-threatening uveitis with no identifiable cause who have LTBI, the recurrence rate of uveitis is greatly reduced with concomitant anti-tubercular therapy (ATT) and immunosuppressive treatment [9–11]. Another important issue, reopened with the introduction of biologics, is obviously the risk of inducing tuberculosis reactivation in patients with severe vision- threatening non-infectious uveitis where systemic corticosteroids and steroid-sparing agents are required. Search for tuberculosis infection is thus an important aspect in the work-up of patients with uveitis, even in low prevalence area in order to prevent reactivation of LTBI [10]. In this chapter, we will review those important aspects of the relation between TB and immunosuppressive (IS) drugs/immunomodulatory treatment (IMT) in uveitis patients.

## 2. Screening in non-infectious uveitis patients for LTBI infection before starting IS or IMT

The mainstay therapy of sight-threatening noninfectious uveitis is based on corticosteroids and immunosuppressive drugs administration. IS drugs are usually restricted to refractory cases and to patients requiring high doses of steroids, in which visual prognosis depends on more aggressive therapeutic approaches. Their long-term use is limited by ocular and systemic side effects.

The introduction of biological agents such as anti- tumor necrosis factor (anti TNF-α), which is a key cytokine in host defense against intracellular infection as Mtb, by regulating the integrity of granuloma where TB is contained, led to the upsurge of TB reactivation [12]. In contrast, none anti-TNF-α targeted biologics like IL-6 inhibitor tocilizumab (TCZ), anti-CD20 rituximab (RTX) and more are not likely associated to any increase risk [13]. To date available TNF alpha booking agents are: infliximab (IFX), adalidumab (ADA), golimumab (GOL), certolizumab peg (CZP) which are monoclonal antibodies directed against TNF alpha, and etanercept (ETN) which is a soluble receptor blocking agent. Several publications reported the effectiveness of anti TNF- drugs in the treatment of uveitis [14, 15]. Anti-TNF treatment had a profound effect on the management of autoimmune vision threatening uveitis with known etiology. ADA is the first licensed anti-TNF treatment for uveitis patients. It is important to emphasize that anti-TNFα agents (infliximab, adalimumab, golimumab) may be more efficient than soluble receptors of TNFα (etanercept) in decreasing the risk of uveitis [16]. But also paradoxical reactions during treatment with a biologic agent, like palmoplantar pustular and psoriasiform reactions, psoriatic arthritis, hidradenitis, inflammatory bowel disease, pyoderma gangrenosum, granulomatous reactions, and vasculitis have subsequently been reported through anecdotal cases, cohort studies, and analysis of drug event databases, showing also that uveitis can flare during anti-TNF-α therapy especially with etanercept [17].

Because of the risk of developing active systemic TB, screening strategies for LTBI detection and preventive therapy for patients undergoing therapy with biological agents have been developed. LTBI is detected either by tuberculin skin test (TST), also named Mantoux test, or by blood-based interferon-gamma release assay (IGRA) including QuantiFERON TB Gold in Tube (QFT). Based on the WHO recommendations, either TST or IGRA are acceptable for LTBI screening [18]. Clinicians may consider, before starting IS, to use IGRA in persons with a history of BCG, but if the index of suspicion of LTBI is high, independently of BCG vaccination, both IGRA and TST may be done, especially prior to initiating anti TNF-α therapy [19]. Recent studies have evaluated the effectiveness of QFT and TST in the screening of arthritis patients and patients with inflammatory bowel disease [20, 21]. Concordance between the two tests was moderate, and it appears lower with immunosuppression. QFT alone may be appropriate in immunosuppressant-naïve patients but both tests should be considered in immunosuppressed patients. In guidelines pertaining to medical immunosuppression, the recommendations for screening varied considerably between the use of TST and IGRA. Concurrent testing with both TST and IGRA was supported by many guidelines [19–23]. Lu et al. conducted a systematic review and meta-analysis to compare the accuracy of IGRAs and TST for the diagnosis of Mtb [24]. IGRAs showed better performance than TST for the diagnosis of the tuberculosis. Data on comparative and cumulative sensitivity and specificity indexes for both tests are detailed in **Table 1**. Cotter and Rosa et al. reported an interesting approach to choose the eligibility for treatment of LTBI after screening with TST and IGRA in immunosuppressed and immunocompetent patients suffering from inflammatory bowel disease, based on a very practical algorithm adapted from Duarte et al. to trace the routes to be followed to decide which patients has LTBI and need tuberculosis treatment according to IGRA and TST [25]. We think that this algorithm can be extrapolated to all patients with inflammatory diseases like uveitis (**Table 2**). Patients with inflammatory diseases who require long-term maintenance medical immunosuppression with a negative screening TST or IGRA may not need further evaluation in the absence of risk factors and/or absence of clinical suspicion for TB in low TB risk countries [19, 21]. Annual evaluation is highly recommended if they live, travel, or work in situations where TB exposure is likely while they continue treatment with biologic agents [23]. It is important to decrease false-positive LTBI testing that may lead to potential toxic antibiotic treatment and result in the unnecessary interruption of biologic therapy. After screening, if either test is positive (TST or IGRA), a chest CT- Scan is mandatory to exclude active pulmonary TB.

LTBI can progress to active TB in 5–10% in subjects who are at higher risk like recent contact, people leaving with HIV, children below 5 years, also an age > 65, immigrants from high TB prevalence countries and candidates of biological

| | QFT-IT | TST |
|---|---|---|
| Sensitivities | 0.842 (95 % CI 0.811-0.870) | 0.665 (CI 0.635-0.693) |
| Specificities | 0.745 (95 % CI 0.715-0.775) | 0.633 (CI 0.605-0.661); |

**Table 1.**
*Data on comparative and cumulative sensitivity and specificity indexes of IGRAs and TST for the diagnosis of tuberculosis.*

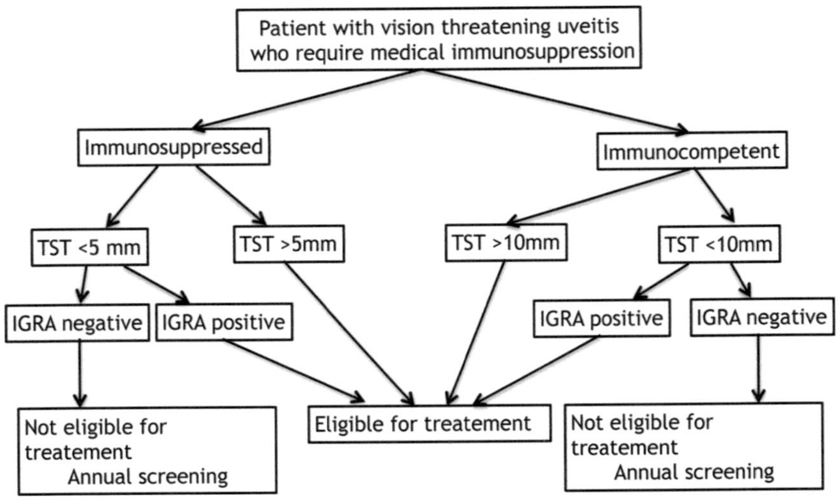


**Table 2.**
*Algorithm for treatment of latent tuberculosis infection in uveitis patients adapted from Duarte et al.*

treatment [18]. When the patient is evaluated, clinicians should also take in account other variables including the host-related TB risk based on age, socioeconomic status, lifestyle, malnutrition, immune-suppression conditions and co-morbidities. The underlying disease itself is also associated with a higher TB risk, with a peak ranging from 2.0 to 8.9 in rheumatoid arthritis patients not receiving biologic therapies, and a lower risk in those with ankylosing spondylitis (AS), psoriatic arthritis (PsA), and psoriasis (Pso) [21–23, 26]. Systemic TB reactivation has rarely been reported as side effect related to Anti-TNF-α therapy in patients with refractory relapsing chronic posterior uveitis [14, 15]. A review of the US Food and Drug Administration (FDA) Adverse Event Reporting System data revealed 70 cases of active TB in 147,000 patients receiving IFX worldwide [22]. Of these, 47 occurred in patients with RA, 18 in those with Crohn's disease, and 5 in people with other types of arthritis, with a median interval of 12 weeks from starting the biologic therapy. The incidence rate of TB was 4 times higher in IFX-treated patients with RA than the estimated incidence in people with RA not receiving biologic therapy. As mentioned, there is an evidence of single biological-related risk as reported by Cantini et al. [10]. The risk is at least 3–4 times higher in patients exposed to monoclonal antibodies IFX and ADA than in those receiving the soluble receptor ETN. Subsequent studies aimed to establish the relative risk (RR) of TB in patients using TNF-α inhibitors (and other biologics) compared to that in the general population. Registries for patients on biologics have provided a valuable resource for studies that aimed to determine the risk of TB associated with these therapies. A French study using the RATIO registry found age- and sex-standardized incidence ratios (SIR) for infliximab, adalimumab, and etanercept of 18.6 (95% CI, 13.4–25.8), 29.3 (95% CI, 20.3–42.4), and 1.8 (95% CI, 0.7–4.3), respectively, compared to that in the general population [27].

Of note, the combined use of anti-TNF agents and traditional DMARDs exposes to a higher risk of TB reactivation in subjects with LTBI compared to patients treated with anti-TNF-α monotherapy. But practicians need to be aware that patients with inflammatory diseases, for which biologics are prescribed, already have an increased risk of TB associated with their immunosuppressed disease state and often also have co-morbidities and additional medications that themselves have an increased risk of TB compared to that of the general population [28]. The risk of TB reactivation in inflammatory patients treated with non-anti-TNF-α target biologics like IL-6 inhibitor tocilizumab (TCZ), anti-CD20 rituximab (RTX) and IL-1 inhibitor anakinra (ANK) and more are not likely associated to any increase risk [13, 29, 30].

Recommendations state that in the case of a diagnosis of LTBI (positive score to an immune diagnostic test (TST or IGRA) and a chest radiograph negative for active TB lesions), active TB prevention with a 6–9-month course of isoniazid is recommended associated to pyridoxine supplementation (vitamin B6), with an average protective effect against TB of 60% during the observation period [31]. There is no clear evidence in the literature concerning the optimal interval between the beginning of the preventive therapy for TB reactivation and biologic therapy [23]. Biologic therapy is suggested to be postponed for at least 1 month thereafter. Therefore, the decision to treat an individual must balance the potential personal benefits against the risk of drug hepatotoxicity and neurotoxicity which is higher in chronic alcoholics, malnourished persons, and pregnant women or healthy individuals (0.2%) due to the inhibitory effect of isoniazid on the function of pyridoxine metabolites. Daily rifampicin alone for 3–4 months compared to placebo has shown a 59% reduction of incident TB [32]. A multi-center clinical trial comparing 4 months of self-administered rifampicin to 9 months of daily isoniazid therapy has been recently completed in 2017. Daily therapy with isoniazid plus rifampicin for 3 months and standard therapy with isoniazid for 6–12 months were equivalent in terms of efficacy and as expected, given the shorter regimen and direct observation, treatment completion was significantly higher in the combination therapy group (82.1% vs. 69.0%). Toxicity was also less reported in the shorter regimen, with fewer individuals taking rifampicin/isoniazid developing drug-related hepatotoxicity [33].

Considering the most frequently used IS and IMT drugs for treatment of non-infectious uveitis, a few specific ophthalmologic reports aims to provide an overview on their use in patients with a recent or past history of systemic serious infection presumably unrelated to their inflammatory eye diseases (IED) [34]. Recently, an expert committee considered assessment and investigation of patients with severe IED initiating immunosuppressive and/or biologic therapy [35]. Infections that may be exacerbated or reactivated as a result of systemic immunosuppressive of biological therapy include: Tuberculosis, hepatitis B virus, hepatitis C virus, HIV and toxoplasmosis. These infection risks should be assessed or exclude before the initiation of such therapy. We keep our focus on risk of TB reactivation in IED patients. Studies regarding this issue are mainly focused on biological therapy, although some studies have indicate the potential risk for developing a TB when using traditional IS agents, particularly MTX [36]. But a significant relationship between the use of MTX and increased incidence of active TB was not established but should be still considered.

While it has been described that If TB develops during anti-TNF-α treatment, it is more likely to be disseminated and extra- pulmonary than are other TB cases. Few reports addressed the occurrence of uveitis tuberculosis development during anti-TNF treatment. A French group reported the uveitis cases occurring in patients with chronic rheumatic diseases, chronic inflammatory intestinal diseases or connective tissue diseases, while treated with disease-modifying anti-rheumatic drugs (DMARDs) and/or biologic therapies. A total of 32 cases of uveitis were reported, and 5 were of infectious origin, 2 toxoplasmosis, 2 herpes virus and 1 tuberculosis [37]. We faced one case of patient with SA and anterior uveitis treated with ADA for years, who developed a panuveitis with choroidal granulomas (**Figure 1**), associated with progressive cough, dyspnea, and pyrexia. A computed tomographic scan

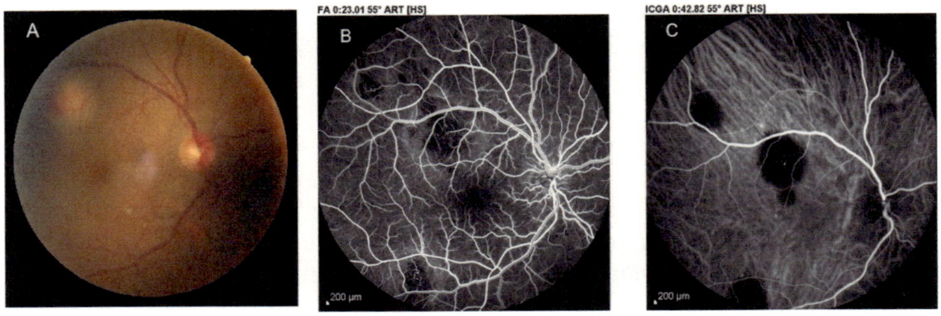


**Figure 1.**
*Bilateral tuberculosis panuveitis developing in a SA patients while under ADA therapy. (A) Eye fundus of the right eye displayed mild vitritis with yellowish deep round infiltrate lesion with discrete subretinal hemorrhage; (B) fluorescein angiogram (FA) at early phase revealed some multifocal hypofluorescent areas, which were easily seen on early stage indocyanin green angiogram (ICG); (C) ICG revealed larger hypofluorescent areas, better delimitated with sharp edges, confirming the choroidal localization of these multiple lesions corresponding to tuberculous granulomas.*

revealed extensive thoracic lymphadenopathy and interstitial shadowing of the lungs. Culture and polymerase chain reaction (PCR) of a mediastinal lymph node biopsy specimen showed acid-fast bacilli.

## 3. Ocular tuberculosis and IMT

There is a great deal of ambiguity in establishing a firm relationship between tuberculosis and ocular inflammation. It's not uncommon, when investigating patients with uveitis, that there is no identifiable systemic or ocular disease and that the only positive test is Mantoux test or QFT associated or not to abnormalities on the chest X-ray. In those patients classically classified as idiopathic uveitis, and treated by immunomodulation, the role of Mtb in disease development has been questioned. On the other hand, the role of immunomodulation in the treatment of well-established tubercular uveitis is also debated.

Severe studies tried to establish a cause/effect relationship between TB and uveitis using some criteria for presumption of tubercular etiology including positive Mantoux test/QFR, healed lesions on the chest X-ray, no other etiology, and suggestive clinical presentation of uveitis [5, 6]. In such patients, the question arises as to whether the uveitis is related to TB or not, leading to the other question of establishing or not ATT.

Intra-ocular TB accounts for 6.9–10.5% of uveitis cases without a known active systemic disease and 1.4–6.8% of patients with active pulmonary disease have concurrent ocular TB [38, 39]. In some patients there is a direct invasion by TB mycobacterium, into local ocular tissues, such as in choroidal granuloma, as evidenced by the histopathological examination of the biopsied involved ocular tissue, smears and cultures of the tissue fluid, and the polymerase chain reaction (PCR). In other patients, there is no clinical evidence to suggest active ocular TB infection. The pathogenesis of uveitis in these patients remains unclear. It is uncertain whether the uveitis is the result of reactivation of LTBI or a hypersensitivity response to Mtb [38, 40]. Bansal proposed guidelines for the diagnosis of intra-ocular TB including a combination of clinical ocular findings, ocular and systemic investigations, exclusion of other etiology and response to ATT [41]. Based on these and their own results, Gupta et al. proposed to classify intra-ocular TB into confirmed, probable, and possible intra-ocular TB [11]. Recently The Collaborative Ocular Tuberculosis Study (COTS)-1 tried to clarify through a multinational retrospective review, what are the suggestive clinical features and approach to diagnosis of patients with tubercular uveitis. The diagnostic criteria for tubercular uveitis used in COTS-1 are developed in **Table 3** [42]. Based on those criteria, we propose a diagram explaining the diagnostic pathways for patients suspected of having TB (**Table 4**). In 2018, they provided in more details the different phenotypes of choroidal involvement in tubercular uveitis, also geographical variations in the phenotypic expression and treatment outcomes. The phenotypic variants reported were serpiginous-like choroiditis (SLC) in 46.1%, choroidal tuberculomas (CTC) in 13.5%, and multifocal choroiditis (MFC) in 9.4%. Other rare phenotypic variants of choroiditis were observed including ampiginous choroiditis (APC) in 9.0% and acute posterior multifocal placoid pigment epitheliopathy (APMPPE) in 3.3% and other indeterminate type of choroiditis in 18.8%. Those varied clinical phenotypes are probably based on the interaction and activity of mycobacterium bacilli and immune system. While SLC was clearly the most prevalent phenotype in the Asia Pacific region, it was less prevalent in the West. Furthermore, APC is a phenotype of choroiditis that is infrequently reported in association with tubercular uveitis [43].

Because TB can be sometimes confined purely to the eye, and as a pauci-bacillary infection, there is a lack of agreed management guidelines among ophthalmologists in establishing the diagnosis of intra-ocular TB. Similarly, there is no agreed consensus between ophthalmologists and other physicians with regards to role of ATT and duration of treatment in cases of isolated intra-ocular TB. Bansal et al. assessed the long-term impact of adding anti-tubercular treatment to the standard anti-inflammatory therapy consisting mostly of corticosteroids in patients with uveitis and evidence of latent or manifest TB. The group speculated that if uveitis was related to hypersensitivity reaction to tubercular antigens attributable to latent TB, the elimination of LTBI would lead to elimination of future recurrences of uveitis in these patients. The administration of anti-tubercular therapy in these patients

| Patients have to satisfy 1 and 2, along with either 3 or 4 for the diagnosis of ocular TB. |
|---|
| **1. Any of the following clinical signs suggestive of ocular tuberculosis including:**<br>a. Anterior uveitis (granulomatous or non-granulomatous) with or without iris nodules or Ciliary body granuloma or<br>b. Intermediate uveitis (granulomatous or non-granulomatous with exudates in the pars plana or peripheral uvea with snow balls) or<br>c. Posterior or Panuveitis - Choroidal tubercle or Choroidal granuloma or Subretinal abscess or Serpiginous-like choroiditis or Retinitis or Retinal vasculitis or Neuroretinitis or Optic neuritis or Endogenous ophthalmitis or Panophthalmitis or Scleritis |
| **2. Exclusion of other uveitic entities where relevant based on clinical manifestations of disease and regional epidemiology** |
| **3. Investigations documenting the mycobacteria or its genome**<br>a. Demonstration of Acid-Fast Bacilli (AFB) by microscopy or culture of M. tuberculosis from ocular fluid<br>b. Positive polymerase chain reaction from ocular fluid for IS 6110 or other conserved sequences in mycobacterial genome<br>c. Evidence of confirmed active pulmonary or extrapulmonary tuberculosis (by microscopic examination or culture of a tissue sample from the affected tissue) |
| **4. Corroborative investigations**<br>a. Positive Mantoux reaction (must be accompanied by information regarding antigen and amount of tuberculin injected, along with institutional practices in interpreting the test)<br>b. Interferon Gamma Release Assay (IGRA) such as Quantiferon TB Gold (must be accompanied by information regarding institutional practices in interpreting the test)<br>c. Evidence of healed or active tuberculosis on chest radiography (must be accompanied by information regarding practices by institution radiologists regarding clinical features that are considered evidence in this regard) |

**Table 3.**
*(COTS)-1 clarify, through a multinational retrospective review, the suggestive clinical features and approach to diagnosis of patients with tubercular (TB) uveitis.*

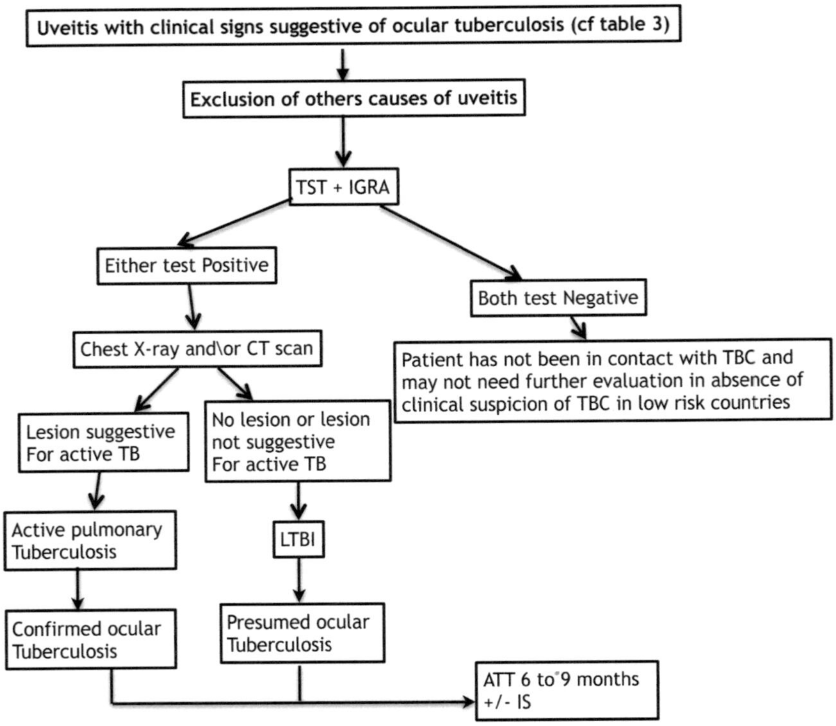


**Table 4.**
*Diagram explaining the diagnostic pathways for patients suspected of having TB.*

substantially reduces recurrences when given along with standard corticosteroid therapy. Corticosteroids may limit damage to ocular tissues caused from delayed type hypersensitivity [41]. The use of ATT to manage presumed ocular tuberculosis is regarded as an effective tool for tubercular uveitis and response to therapy can be a good surrogate for diagnosis of presumed ocular tuberculosis.

A case control study conducted by Chee et al. on patients with uveitis with evidence of latent TB and no other underlying disease, who were treated with ATT for more than 9 months duration, were approximately 11 times less likely to develop recurrence of inflammation compared with patients who had not received ATT. This association was independent of potential confounders such as demographics, classification of uveitis and corticosteroid therapy. On the other hand, patients who were treated with ATT for <6 months or 6–9 months duration did have a reduction in recurrence, but this was not statistically significant [39]. The Collaborative Ocular Tuberculosis Study (COTS)-1 group also reported the role of ATT in the management of patients with TB uveitis from a multinational cohort and explore potential correlations of clinical features with treatment response. A low treatment failure rate was reported in patients with TB uveitis treated with ATT. On multivariate regression analysis, they showed that the presence of choroidal involvement with vitreous haze and snowballs in patients with panuveitis was associated with a higher risk of recurrence. Concerning the addition of corticosteroids to ATT, their results suggests that patients treated with corticosteroids may have had poorer outcomes than those who were not [42]. Effectively, the possible beneficial effect of immunomodulation in association of ATT in the management of tubercular uveitis is still debated. A recent meta analyze was conducted on 37 articles to assess the effect of ATT associated or not to IMT on ocular outcome of patients with presumed ocular TB. The meta-analysis revealed that 84% of the patients receiving ATT showed non-recurrence of inflammation during the follow-up period. A successful outcome was observed in 85% of patients treated with ATT alone; in 82% of patients treated with ATT and systemic steroids and in 85% of patients treated with ATT and systemic steroids and immunomodulators. It was not possible to conclude which regimen was the best to control ocular inflammation [44–46].

## 4. Conclusion

The link between tuberculosis, uveitis and immunosuppression are important and complex. First, patients with inflammatory diseases treated with IMT agents, including noninfectious uveitis patients, are at risk to develop active tuberculosis, including ocular tuberculosis. Secondly, many data suggest that Mtb might play a role in disease development of idiopathic uveitis in LTBI patients and that ATT must be considered in such cases. Finally, inflammatory and immune reaction are likely to play a role during ocular tuberculosis and immunomodulation has a beneficial effect.

In summary, we have to keep in mind that the main concern of TB screening for ophthalmologist is to avoid systemic TB reactivation in front of a sight threatening uveitis with known etiology destined to IS/IMT. But when facing an idiopathic uveitis under IS/IMT, there is another risks which has to be considered, the risk of ocular TB misdiagnosis with a non- or partial response to immunosuppressive treatment. Introduction of ATT in those cases will control inflammation, will help to discontinue most IMT and will prevent recurrences.

## Author details

François Willermain[1,2], Laure Caspers[1], Weber Celia[1,2] and Dorine Makhoul[1,2]*

1 Department of Ophthalmology, CHU Saint-Pierre, Université Libre de Bruxelles, Brussels, Belgium

2 Department of Ophthalmology, CHU Brugmann, Université Libre de Bruxelles, Brussels, Belgium

*Address all correspondence to: domakhoul@gmail.com

## References


[1] Wirth T, Hildebrand F, Allix-Béguec C, et al. Origin, spread and demography of the Mycobacterium tuberculosis complex. PLoS Pathogen. 2008;**4**:e100160

[2] Dye C, Scheele S, Dolin P, Pathania V, Raviglione MC. Consensus statement. Global burden of tuberculosis: Estimated incidence, prevalence, and mortality by country. WHO global surveillance and monitoring project. JAMA. 1999;**282**:677-686

[3] Lonnroth K, Raviglione M. Global epidemiology of tuberculosis: Prospects for control. Seminars in Respiratory and Critical Care Medicine. 2008;**29**:481-491

[4] Maartens G, Wilkinson RJ. Tuberculosis. Lancet. 2007;**370**:2030-2043

[5] Gupta V, Gupta A, Rao NR. Intraocular tuberculosis—An update. Survey of Ophthalmology. 2007;**52**:561-587

[6] Cunningham ET. TB or not TB ? The perennial question. The British Journal of Ophthalmology. 2001;**85**:127-129

[7] Agrawal R, Gupta B, González-López JJ, et al. Spectrum of choroidal involvement in presumed ocular tuberculosis: Report from a population with low endemic setting for tuberculosis. Ocular Immunology and Inflammation. 2017;**25**(1):97-104

[8] Agrawal R, Gunasekeran DV, Grant R, et al. Clinical features and outcomes of patients with tubercular uveitis treated with antitubecular therapy in the collaborative ocular tuberculosis study (COTS)-1. JAMA Ophthalmology. DOI: 10.1001/jamaophthalmol.2017.4485. 2017.10.26

[9] Agrawal R, Gupta B, Gonzalez-Lopez JJ, et al. The role of anti-tubercular therapy in patients with presumed ocular tuberculosis. Ocular Immunology and Inflammation. 2015;**23**(1):40-46

[10] Cantini F, Niccoli L, Goletti D. Adalimumab, etanercept, infliximab, and the risk of tuberculosis: Data from clinical trials, national registries, and postmarketing surveillance. The Journal of Rheumatology. Supplement. 2014;**91**:47-55

[11] Bansal R, Gupta A, Gupta V, et al. Role of anti-tubercular therapy in uveitis with latent/manifest tuberculosis. American Journal of Ophthalmology. 2008;**146**(5):772-779

[12] Shobha V, Chandrashekara S, Rao V, Desai A, Jois R, Dharmanand BG, et al. Biologics and risk of tuberculosis in autoimmune rheumatic diseases: A real-world clinical experience from India. International Journal of Rheumatic Diseases. 2018

[13] Cantini F, Nannini C, Niccoli L, Petrone L, Ippolito G, Goletti D. Risk of tuberculosis reactivation in patients with rheumatoid arthritis, ankylosing spondylitis, and psoriatic arthritis receiving non-anti-TNF-targeted biologics. Mediators of Inflammation. 2017;**2017**:8909834

[14] Calvo-Río V, Blanco R, Beltrán E, Sánchez-Bursón J, Mesquida M, Adán A, et al. Anti-TNF-α therapy in patients with refractory uveitis due to Behçet's disease: A 1-year follow-up study of 124 patients. Rheumatology (Oxford, England). 2014 Dec;**53**(12):2223-2231

[15] Joseph A, Raj D, Dua HS, Powell PT, Lanyon PC, Powell RJ. Infliximab in the treatment of refractory posterior uveitis. Ophthalmology. 2003 Jul;**110**(7):1449-1453

[16] Mitulescu TC, Trandafir M, Dimăncescu MG, Ciuluvică RC, Popescu

V, Predețeanu D, et al. Advances in the treatment of uveitis in patients with spondyloarthritis—Is it the time for biologic therapy? Romanian Journal of Ophthalmology. 2018;**62**(2):114-122. Review

[17] Puig L. Paradoxical reactions: Anti-tumor necrosis factor alpha agents, ustekinumab, secukinumab, ixekizumab, and others. Current Problems in Dermatology

[18] Getahun H, Chaisson RE, Raviglione M. Latent mycobacterium tuberculosis infection. The New England Journal of Medicine. 2015;**373**(12):1179-1180

[19] Goletti D, Petrone L, Ippolito G, Niccoli L, Nannini C, Cantini F. Preventive therapy for tuberculosis in rheumatological patients undergoing therapy with biological drugs. Expert Review of Anti-Infective Therapy. 2018;**16**(6):501-512

[20] Lee H, Park HY, Jeon K, Jeong BH, Hwang JW, Lee J, et al. QuantiFERON-TB gold in-tube assay for screening arthritis patients for latent tuberculosis infection before starting anti-tumor necrosis factor treatment. PLoS One. 2015;**10**(3):e0119260

[21] Mantzaris GJ, Tsironikos D, Tzanetakou X, Grispou E, Karatzas P, Kalogeropoulos I, et al. The impact of immunosuppressive therapy on QuantiFERON and tuberculin skin test for screening of latent tuberculosis in patients with inflammatory bowel disease scheduled for anti-TNF therapy. Scandinavian Journal of Gastroenterology. 2015;**50**(12):1451-1455

[22] Cantini F, Nannini C, Niccoli L, Iannone F, Delogu G, Garlaschi G, et al. Guidance for the management of patients with latent tuberculosis infection requiring biologic therapy in rheumatology and dermatology clinical practice. Autoimmunity Reviews. 2015;**14**(6):503-509

[23] Iannone F, Cantini F, Lapadula G. Diagnosis of latent tuberculosis and prevention of reactivation in rheumatic patients on biologic therapy: The international recommendations. The Journal of Rheumatology. Supplement. 2014;**91**:41-46

[24] Lu P, Chen X, Zhu L, Yang H. Interferon-gamma release assays for the diagnosis of tuberculosis: A systematic review and meta-analysis. Lung. 2016;**194**(3):447-458

[25] Duarte R, Campainha S, Cotter J, Rosa B, Varela P, Correia A, et al. Position paper on tuberculosis screening in patients with immune mediated inflammatory diseases candidates for biological therapy. Acta Reumatológica Portuguesa. 2012;**37**(3):253-259

[26] Wong SH, Gao Q, Tsoi KK, Wu WK, Tam LS, Lee N, et al. Effect of immunosuppressive therapy on interferon γ release assay for latent tuberculosis screening in patients with autoimmune diseases: A systematic review and meta-analysis. Thorax. 2016;**71**(1):64-72

[27] Dobler CC. Biologic agents and tuberculosis. Microbiology Spectrum. 2016;**4**(6)

[28] Lorenzetti R, Zullo A, Ridola L, Diamanti AP, Laganà B, Gatta L, et al. Higher risk of tuberculosis reactivation when anti-TNF is combined with immunosuppressive agents: A systematic review of randomized controlled trials. Annals of Medicine. 2014;**46**:547-554

[29] Payet S, Soubrier M, Perrodeau E, Bardin T, Cantagrel A, Combe B, et al. Efficacy and safety of rituximab in elderly patients with rheumatoid arthritis enrolled in a French Society of Rheumatology registry. Arthritis Care and Research. 2014;**66**:1289-1295

[30] Cantarini L, Lopalco G, Caso F, Costa L, Iannone F, Lapadula G, et al.

Effectiveness and tuberculosis-related safety profile of interleukin-1 blocking agents in the management of Behçet's disease. Autoimmunity Reviews. 2015;**14**:1-9

[31] International Union Against Tuberculosis Committee on Prophylaxis. Efficacy of various durations of isoniazid preventive therapy for tuberculosis: Five years of follow-up in the IUAT trial. Bulletin of the World Health Organization. 1982;**60**(4):555-564

[32] Menzies D. Randomized clinical trial comparing RIF vs. INH for LTBI treatment-effectiveness. 2016. NCT00931736

[33] Ena J, Valls V. Short-course therapy with rifampin plus isoniazid, compared with standard therapy with isoniazid, for latent tuberculosis infection: A meta-analysis. Clinical Infectious Diseases. 2005;**40**(5):670-676

[34] Cordero-Coma M, Salazar-Méndez R, Yilmaz T. Treatment of severe non-infectious uveitis in high-risk conditions (part 2): Systemic infections; management and safety issues. Expert Opinion on Drug Safety. 2015;**14**(9):1353-1371

[35] Wakefield D, McCluskey P, Wildner G, Thurau S, Carr G, Chee SP, et al. Inflammatory eye disease: Pre-treatment assessment of patients prior to commencing immunosuppressive and biologic therapy: Recommendations from an expert committee. Autoimmunity Reviews. 2017;**16**(3):213-222

[36] Zorlu M, Kiskac M, Karatoprak C, et al. Pott's disease and hypercalcemia in a patient with rheumatoid arthritis receiving methotrexate monotherapy. Indian Journal of Pharmacology. 2013;**45**(6):631-633

[37] Cabane L, Baillif S, Baldin B, Breuil V, Euller-Ziegler L, Tieulié N. Uveitis treated with biotherapy and/or DMARD: Analysis from the French Pharmacovigilance Study Base. Journal Français d'Ophtalmologie. 2018;**41**(4):350-356

[38] Alvarez GG, Roth VR, Hodge W. Ocular tuberculosis: Diagnostic and treatment challenges. International Journal of Infectious Diseases. 2009;**13**(4):432-435

[39] Ang M, Hedayatfar A, Wong W, et al. Duration of anti-tubercular therapy in uveitis associated with latent tuberculosis: A case-control study. The British Journal of Ophthalmology. 2012;**96**(3):332-336

[40] Helm CJ, Holland GN. Ocular tuberculosis. Survey of Ophthalmology. 1993;**38**:229-256

[41] Bansal R, Gupta A, Gupta V, et al. Tubercular serpiginous-like choroiditis presenting as multifocal serpiginoid choroiditis. Ophthalmology. 2012;**119**(11):2334-2342

[42] Agrawal R, Gunasekeran DV, Grant R, Agarwal A, Kon OM, Nguyen QD, et al. Clinical features and outcomes of patients with tubercular uveitis treated with antitubercular therapy in the collaborative ocular tuberculosis study (COTS)-1. JAMA Ophthalmology. 2017;**135**(12):1318-1327

[43] Agrawal R, Gunasekeran DV, Agarwal A, Carreño E, Aggarwal K, Gupta B, et al. The collaborative ocular tuberculosis study (COTS)-1: A multinational description of the spectrum of choroidal involvement in 245 patients with tubercular uveitis. Ocular Immunology and Inflammation. 2018;**29**:1-1

[44] Kee AR, Gonzalez-Lopez JJ, Al-Hity A, Gupta B, Lee CS, Gunasekeran

DV, et al. Anti-tubercular therapy for intraocular tuberculosis: A systematic review and meta-analysis. Survey of Ophthalmology. 2016;**61**(5):628-653

[45] Bajema KL, Pakzad-Vaezi K, Hawn T, Pepple KL. Tuberculous uveitis: Association between anti-tuberculous therapy and clinical response in a non-endemic country. Journal of Ophthalmic Inflammation and Infection. 2017;**7**(1):19

[46] Tomkins-Netzer O, Leong BCS, Zhang X, Lightman S, McCluskey PJ, Sydney-London Latent Ocular TB Study Group. Effect of antituberculous therapy on uveitis associated with latent tuberculosis. American Journal of Ophthalmology. 2018;**190**:164-170

Section 3

# Advances in Therapeutic Strategies for Uveitis

Chapter 6

# A Novel Ocular Drug Delivery System of Dexamethasone Sodium Phosphate for Noninfectious Uveitis Treatment

*Kongnara Papangkorn, John W. Higuchi, Balbir Brar and William I. Higuchi*

## Abstract

Treatment of anterior uveitis commonly requires 6–8 times daily administration of eye drops, which often leads to poor patient compliance. The treatment of intermediate and posterior uveitis is restricted to either oral medications with significant systemic side effects or local invasive methods, which are more expensive and associated with the development of ocular complications. There is an unmet need for a new drug delivery system that addresses these challenges. DSP-Visulex is a noninvasive drug delivery system that administers dexamethasone sodium phosphate by passive diffusion through the limbal sclera into the interior of the eye utilizing the transscleral pathway. Once-a-week administration of DSP-Visulex treatment regimens (i.e., 1–5 doses per month) has shown to be safe and efficacious for noninfectious uveitis in animal models including anterior uveitis, posterior uveitis, and/or panuveitis. In a clinical study of anterior uveitis, the DSP-Visulex treatments also have been shown to be safe and well tolerated and their efficacy (administered on days 1, 3, 8, and 15 with an optional treatment on Day 22) was comparable to that of the daily prednisolone acetate drops.

**Keywords:** noninvasive, ocular drug delivery, dexamethasone, safety and efficacy, topical treatment, uveitis

## 1. Introduction

Uveitis represents a group of intraocular inflammatory disorders which may result in significant visual loss and is responsible for approximately 10–15% of blindness in the USA [1–4]. The annual prevalence of uveitis ranges from 58 to 115 cases per 100,000 persons [4–6]. Anterior uveitis is the most common anatomic location representing approximately 70% of all the uveitis cases in the USA [4–6]. Although posterior and panuveitis are far less common, they owe a greater consequence in blindness [7].

Dexamethasone sodium phosphate (DSP) is a highly water-soluble form of dexamethasone. DSP undergoes rapid hydrolysis to form dexamethasone (DEX) in plasma [8] and ocular tissues [9]. Both DEX and DSP have been used for the treatment of a wide variety of ocular inflammation conditions such as keratitis, blepharitis, iritis, conjunctivitis, uveitis, macular edema, and post-operative eye surgery [10]. There are a number of dosage forms of DEX and DSP for ocular treatments including eye drops, ointments, oral tablets, intraocular injections, and intravitreal implants. Current topical methods, however, cannot deliver drugs to the posterior segment of the eye effectively and their practice has been limited to treating anterior eye conditions [11–13]. Eye drops often yield poor patient compliance due to the required adherence to frequent administration [14]. The posterior segment of the eye can be treated systemically but significant whole-body adverse effects are major concerns [12]. Invasive methods, such as periocular injections, intravitreal injections, or intravitreal implants (e.g., Ozurdex®, Retisert®, Iluvien®, etc.), are effective but the cost of administration is high. They also involve a number of potential serious risks including retinal detachment, endophthalmitis, increased intraocular pressure (IOP), and cataractogenesis [15–18]. There is an unmet need for a new drug delivery system that can address such challenges.

Recent publications suggest that treating back-of-the-eye diseases using topical administration is feasible [19–24]. For topically administered drugs, the transscleral pathway can be a route for a drug molecule to reach posterior eye tissues [25–31]. A fluorophotometry study in live rabbits suggests that once drug is placed intrasclerally, there is an active, convective flow carrying drug molecules through the suprachoroidal space to the retina-choroid region at the back of the eye [32]. To administer drug through this pathway effectively, a high drug concentration on the sclera is an ideal prerequisite. This is because drug diffuses across eye tissues by concentration gradients as described by Fick's first law of diffusion: $\text{Flux} = PA(C_1 - C_2)$. Flux is the amount of drug that passes through a membrane per period of time (mg/sec). P is the permeability coefficient of the permeant (cm/sec), A is the surface area ($cm^2$) over which diffusion is taking place, and $(C_1 - C_2)$ is the difference in concentration (mg/mL) of the permeant across the membrane for the direction of flow from $C_1$ to $C_2$. Thus, a high concentration in the applicator ($C_1$) may significantly increase flux. However, the current topical ophthalmic products have failed to utilize this pathway effectively because of the short retention time at the site of application and the low drug concentration used in its formulation.

## 2. Visulex-P, a novel ocular drug delivery system

Visulex-P is a noninvasive ocular drug delivery system that can be used to administer drug topically through the limbal sclera into the interior of the eye utilizing the transscleral pathway [33, 34]. It is a passive diffusion-base technology developed by Aciont Inc. designed to facilitate the drug molecule entering primarily through the conjunctiva-scleral surface and minimize the drug clearance from tearing and drainage into the nasolacrimal duct. In addition, Visulex-P enables an ophthalmic application of a high drug concentration, which may expedite the passive drug diffusion through the transscleral pathway without significant ocular toxicity [34]. DSP is suitable for Visulex-P because of its high water solubility, enabling a high drug-driving force, and its high potency with respect to prednisolone acetate on a molar basis. In this chapter, the combination of this high DSP-concentration solution instilled into the Visulex-P applicator is referred to as DSP-Visulex.

## 3. DSP-Visulex administration

DSP-Visulex may be administered to a patient in a general clinical setting by a physician, nurse, or trained technician, and in some cases, it may be

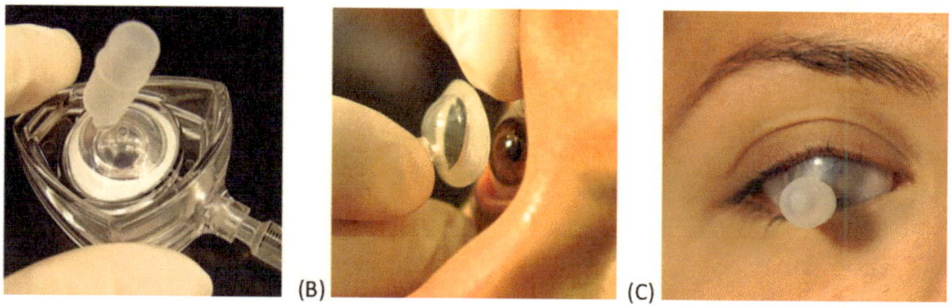

(A) (B) (C)

**Figure 1.**
*(A) Dexamethasone sodium phosphate (DSP) solution is being loaded into Visulex applicator through a drug loader. (B) DSP-Visulex is being applied onto the eye. (C) DSP-Visulex is on the eye where the sponge is in contact with the eye on the sclera and the surface area of the sponge is approximately 150 mm$^2$.*

self-administered at home. The Visulex applicator resembles the handling and feel of a scleral lens which is a type of contact lens worn throughout the day by the patient who is suffering from corneal shape disorders or injuries to the eye. The details and video of DSP-Visulex administration follow:

There are a few steps in DSP-Visulex administration (**Figure 1**). Proparacaine (0.5%), a topical anesthetic agent, is first applied to the patient's eye(s). The DSP solution (250 μL) is loaded into the Visulex-P applicator with the drug loader just prior to application. The drug-loaded applicator (DSP-Visulex) is removed carefully from the loader. The DSP-Visulex is then gently placed directly onto the sclera while the care giver holds the patient's upper and lower eyelids open. The Visulex applicator is checked to ensure that it remains centered on the eye and does not make contact with the cornea throughout the treatment duration. After the treatment duration (e.g., 5 minutes), the Visulex applicator is carefully removed by squeezing the entire bulb to release the vacuum while lifting the applicator up from the eye. The DSP-Visulex is discarded after this single administration and is not reused. The DSP-Visulex administration for animal studies was similar to that in the clinical study except each animal was placed in a restrainer to limit movement during the DSP-Visulex administration.

## 4. Two main factors of DSP-Visulex affecting the amount of drug in the rabbit eye

Both the DSP concentration and the treatment duration of DSP-Visulex correlate with the total amount of drug in the eye [35]. After single applications of DSP-Visulex for 5, 10, or 20 minutes and for all DSP concentrations, significant amounts (i.e., 56–760 μg) of DSP were found in the eye (**Figure 2**). When qualitatively comparing both factors with respect to the whole eye, it appears that the relative increase in DSP-Visulex concentration affected the ocular tissue concentrations more than the treatment duration.

For instance, in **Figure 2** at the 5-minute application time, when the DSP concentration is increased from 4 to 15%, which is about a factor of 4, the total amount of the drug in the eye increased by about fivefold from 56 μg to 288 μg, but when the application time is increased from 5 to 20 minutes, which is also a factor of 4, the total amount of the drug in the eye increased by only twofold from 56 μg to 104 μg. This relationship appears to hold for sclera, conjunctiva, cornea, and anterior chamber (AC), but is more subtle for vitreous, retina-choroid, and lens (discussed in a later section).

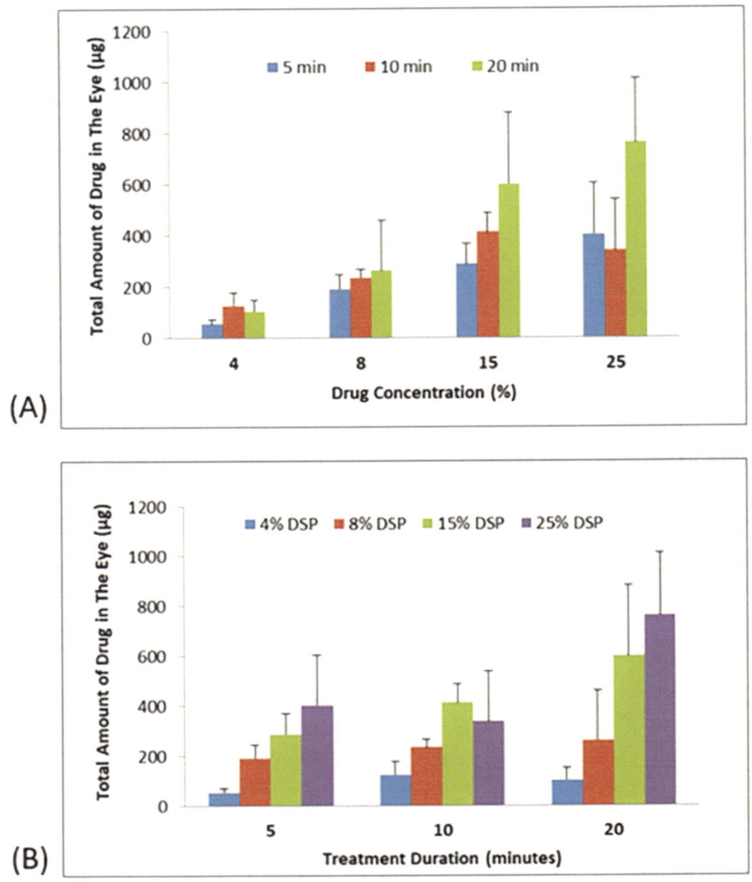


**Figure 2.**
*(A) Effect of drug concentration on total amount of drug in the eye. (B) Effect of drug concentration on total amount of drug in the eye.*

## 5. Drug distribution in the eye after DSP-Visulex application

The ocular drug distribution study of DSP-Visulex in rabbit illustrates the potential for the noninvasive delivery of DSP into the eye tissues from anterior to posterior section [35]. After single applications of DSP-Visulex for 5, 10, or 20 minutes and for all DSP concentrations, significant amounts of DSP and some DEX were found in all eye tissues. A typical rank order of DSP amounts in the eye tissues is sclera, conjunctiva, cornea, retina-choroid, anterior chamber, vitreous, and lens. The total amount of drugs in each tissue except vitreous and lens appears to be correlated well with the DSP concentration and application time of DSP-Visulex.

In **Table 1**, the concentration of DSP in each tissue is calculated in µg/g and summarized for potential efficacy evaluation of DSP-Visulex and the concentration of 1 µg/g or higher in the tissue is considered a potential therapeutic level [35]. After a single administration of DSP-Visulex, with exception of the lens, DSP found in most of the ocular tissues including cornea, sclera, conjunctiva, retina-choroid, and anterior chamber was significantly higher than the target level of 1 µg/g in all of the DSP-Visulex regimens tested in the study. DSP concentrations in the vitreous were around or slightly above 1 µg/g in most cases except for the 5-minute 4% DSP application. The typical order of concentration of DSP in ocular tissues, from high to low, was: cornea > sclera >

| Dose | Tissue (mean ± SD, μg/g) | | | | | | |
|---|---|---|---|---|---|---|---|
| | Cornea | Anterior chamber | Lens | Vitreous | Retina-choroid | Sclera | Conjunctiva |
| 4% DSP, 5 min | 108±74 | 14±4 | 0±0 | 0±1 | 18±16 | 59±25 | 33±29 |
| 4% DSP, 10min | 216 ± 86 | 11 ± 8 | 2 ± 0 | 2 ± 1 | 59 ± 86 | 131 ± 52 | 56 ± 14 |
| 4% DSP, 20min | 147 ± 75 | 12 ± 4 | 3 ± 1 | 1 ± 1 | 24 ± 7 | 154 ± 49 | 49 ± 26 |
| 8% DSP, 5 min | 288±73 | 23±3 | 13±0 | 5±1 | 74±23 | 233±53 | 84±36 |
| 8% DSP, 10 min | 459±148 | 23±9 | 0±0 | 2±1 | 63±61 | 314±74 | 104=33 |
| 8% DSP, 20 min | 567 ± 397 | 56 ± 54 | 14 ± 24 | 6 ± 8 | 54 ± 38 | 306 ± 207 | 113 ± 58 |
| 15% DSP, 5 min | 367±118 | 18±3 | 5±0 | 5±3 | 182±176 | 328±60 | 150=26 |
| 15% DSP, 10 min | 467 ± 173 | 43 ± 11 | 17 ± 1 | 7 ± 1 | 113 ± 32 | 512 ± 54 | 222 ± 45 |
| 15% DSP, 20 min | 1128 ± 521 | 89 ± 42 | 13 ± 3 | 12 ± 3 | 351 ± 275 | 615 ± 336 | 287= 94 |
| 25% DSP, 5 min | 714±252 | 39±17 | 6±1 | 6±3 | 114±82 | 452±214 | 221±126 |
| 25% DSP, 10 min | 512 ± 327 | 35 ± 32 | 1 ± 1 | 4 ± 4 | 60 ± 77 | 429 ± 231 | 184 ± 109 |
| 25% DSP, 20 min | 2225 ± 886 | 169 ± 67 | 13 ± 4 | 9 ± 4 | 207 ± 101 | 731 ± 189 | 347 ± 107 |

**Table 1.**
*Dexamethasone sodium phosphate-equivalent concentrations in ocular tissues.*

conjunctiva > retina-choroid > anterior chamber > lens > vitreous. The drug concentration in the ocular tissues (except lens and vitreous) correlated well with both increasing DSP concentration in the Visulex system and treatment duration.

Although the dynamics of aqueous flow and clearance in the eye are complex, the ocular drug distribution results are in line with an anticipated concentration gradient pattern arising from the outer eye tissues like sclera and conjunctiva, which were adjacent to the DSP drug reservoir and received the most drug, to the innermost tissues like the vitreous humor and lens that received much lesser amounts. Additionally, it should be noted this study was limited only to one time point, which was immediately after the DSP-Visulex application. More study time points should yield further understanding of the pharmacokinetic profiles of DSP administered by the DSP-Visulex including drug distribution, onset, duration of action, and half-life of the drug in the eye tissues.

Comparing the DSP-Visulex in rabbit to periocular injections and oral administration in human [36], the DSP concentration in rabbit retina-choroid after a single administration of DSP-Visulex ranged from 18 to 351 μg/g whereas the estimated maximum DEX concentration in the subretinal fluid in patients after an oral dose of DEX (7.5 mg), a peribulbar injection (5 mg), and a subconjunctival injection (2.5 mg) was 12, 82, and 359 ng/mL, respectively [36]. When qualitatively comparing DSP-Visulex application in rabbit to the topical DSP eye drop (i.e., 1 drop of 0.1% DSP every 1.5 hours for a total of 10 or 11 drops) in human [37], the concentration of DSP in the vitreous of rabbit from DSP-Visulex is much higher: the $C_{max}$ in human vitreous from the DSP eye drop was 1 ng/mL while most DSP-Visulex regimens yield ~1 μg/mL or more in the vitreous of rabbit. While such indirect comparisons of the DSP-Visulex data in rabbit with the pharmacokinetic studies in human may be unavailing, these at least illustrate the potential significance of the DSP-Visulex approach.

## 6. Systemic exposure after single application of DSP-Visulex

A toxicokinetic study in rabbit suggests that DSP was rapidly absorbed into the systemic circulation after the DSP-Visulex application [35]. The plasma concentrations of DSP and DEX after single applications of DSP-Visulex are shown in **Figure 3**. $T_{max}$ of DSP was reached at the first blood draw (5 minutes after DSP-Visulex application), whereas $T_{max}$ of DEX was reached later at 30 minutes. The maximum plasma concentration ($C_{max}$) of both DSP and DEX increased with increasing DSP concentration and with longer application time. Within 24 hours, the drug plasma concentrations of all groups were approaching or under the lowest detection limit of 1 ng/mL.

For the purpose of assessing the systemic exposure of total corticosteroid after DSP-Visulex application, the DSP and DEX plasma concentrations were combined and calculated as DSP equivalent. The DSP equivalent is defined as the sum of DSP and DEX in gram equivalents, with 392.5 g of DEX equivalent to 516.4 g of DSP. The key toxicokinetic parameters are presented in **Table 2**. The systemic half-life of the drug in the rabbit is approximately 2–3 hours. $C_{max}$ and AUC increased with increased concentration of DSP and increased application time. Similar to the eye results, the concentration seems to have more effect on the systemic exposure than application duration. For example, when the DSP concentration was increased from 4 to 15%, which is about a factor of 4, the $C_{max}$ increased about eightfold from 148 μg to 1188 μg, but when the application time increased from 5 to 20 minutes, which is also a factor of 4, the total amount of the drug in the eye increased only fourfold from 148 μg to 795 μg. This was also the case with AUC. The increase in concentration from 4 to 15% increased the AUC by a factor of 4, whereas the increase in the application time from 5 to 20 minutes increased the AUC only by a factor of 2.

To express the results of systemic DSP exposure in rabbit in human perspective, $C_{max}$ values of DSP in human were estimated and are presented in **Table 2**. The estimations were based on $C_{max}$ data from intravenous (IV) injections in both rabbit [38] and human [39]: An IV injection of 1 mg DSP yields a $C_{max}$ of 786 ng/mL in rabbit and 10.5 ng/mL in human. Accordingly, these results suggest that at a given dose of DSP,

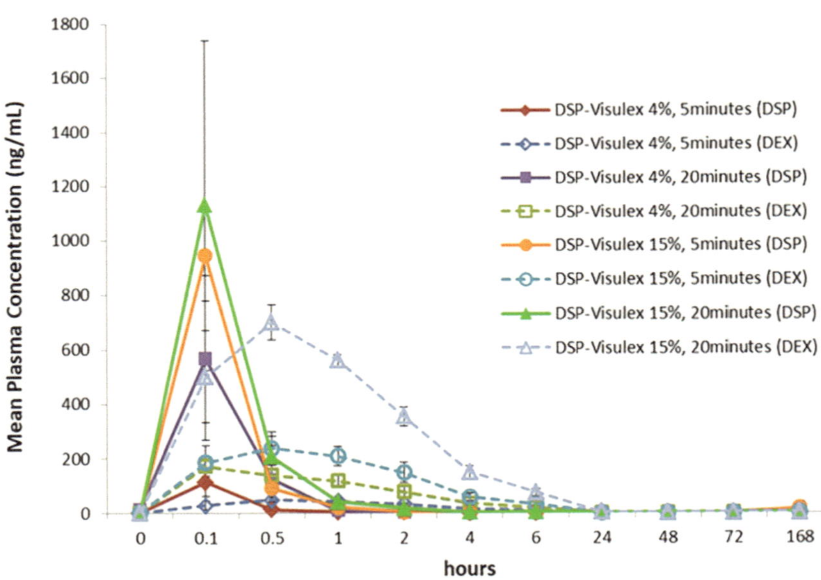


**Figure 3.**
*Mean plasma concentration of DSP (solid line) and DEX (dot line) following single administration of DSP-Visulex at predose, 5, 30, 60, 120, 240, and 360 minutes, and 24, 48, 72, and 168 hours. To reveal all pharmacokinetic data, all the graphs were not plotted in a linear time scale on the x-axis.*

| Dose | $C_{max}$ (ng/mL) | $t_{1/2}$ (h) | AUC (ng*h/mL) | Estimated $C_{max}$ in Human (ng/mL) |
|---|---|---|---|---|
| 4% DSP, 5 min | 148± 71 | 3.1 ± 2.2 | 418 ± 93 | 2 ± 1 |
| 4% DSP, 20 min | 795 ± 344 | 2.3 ± 0.6 | 996 ± 144 | 11 ± 5 |
| 15% DSP, 5 min | 1188 ± 306 | 1.7 ± 0.9 | 1595 ± 418 | 16 ± 4 |
| 15% DSP, 20 min | 1844 ± 664 | 2.7 ± 0.3 | 3779 ± 472 | 25 ± 9 |

**Table 2.**
*Dexamethasone sodium phosphate-equivalent concentrations in plasma.*

the $C_{max}$ of DSP for rabbit is approximately 75 times higher than that for human. The estimated $C_{max}$ values in human of the lowest dose (4% DSP, 5 minutes) and the highest dose of DSP-Visulex (15% DSP, 20 minutes) are 2 and 25 ng/mL, respectively. In addition, the estimated $C_{max}$ values in human in the range of 2–25 ng/mL may be supported by an ocular iontophoretic delivery of dexamethasone phosphate (4%w/v) in uveitis patients, which showed the plasma $C_{max}$ of dexamethasone in the range of 2–10 ng/mL [40]. This is because the ocular iontophoresis delivered approximately the same order of magnitude of dexamethasone phosphate to the rabbit ocular tissues as DSP-Visulex [35], it is reasonable to speculate that the systemic drug exposure in human of DSP-Visulex would be in the same order of magnitude as the ocular iontophoresis.

When compared to the plasma $C_{max}$ from a single application of DSP-Visulex to the literature $C_{max}$ from a single IVT injection, a single topical eye drop, an oral tablet, a single peribulbar injection, and a single subconjunctival injection [41], it suggests that DSP-Visulex may have a higher systemic exposure than eye drops and IVT injections but less than oral and periocular injections (i.e., peribulbar injection and subconjunctival injection).

## 7. Ocular toxicity of DSP-Visulex in animal

A 12-week toxicity study of DSP-Visulex at 4, 8, 15, and 25% suggests that multiple treatments of DSP-Visulex are well tolerated [35]. The ocular findings observed in treated eyes from the study (i.e., 20-minute treatment duration of DSP-Visulex) were conjunctival injection, chemosis discharge, and corneal haze. These ocular findings were transient and mild in nature. No abnormalities or signs of ocular toxicity were observed in untreated eyes. The only frequent ocular adverse event was conjunctival injection, which appeared to resolve within a week. This sign of irritation correlates with increasing DSP concentration. Some accumulations of conjunctival injection were observed in the high concentration formulations (i.e., 15 and 25% DSP) after 2 months into the weekly treatment regimen. The tonicity of the DSP formulation may have played a role in the conjunctival irritation. The persistence and severity of the conjunctival irritation were found to be much lower in the 4 and 8% DSP formulations (i.e., isotonic formulation) compared to the 15 and 25% formulation (i.e., hypertonic formulation). It may be noted that conjunctival injection, which is also known as conjunctival hyperemia or conjunctival erythema, is a common side effect found among FDA-approved corticosteroid ophthalmic solutions including prednisolone, dexamethasone, and difluprednate. A temporary corneal haze was found in one rabbit when the placement of DSP-Visulex is placed off center. This is an adverse effect that can be avoided by checking whether the DSP reservoir has any direct contact with the cornea while in position during treatment.

As for the histopathology after multiple treatments of DSP-Visulex for 12 weeks, all eyes were considered to be morphologically normal, except one treated eye in the 8% DSP group showed mild chronic inflammation at the limbus of the cornea. Besides this one eye, there were no significant findings with any ocular tissue examined: no edema or congestion of conjunctiva, ciliary body, or cornea was observed in any group; no neovascularization on the cornea was found; and no inflammation in conjunctiva, cornea, anterior chamber, trabecular meshwork, iris, ciliary body, vitreous, choroid, and retina tissues and no test article changes were identified.

There were no significant weight changes in the 4 or 8% DSP-treated rabbits. However, the animals in the 15 and 25% DSP groups showed trends of decreasing body weight. Although only the 25% DSP group showed statistically significant reduction in body weight, the consistent decline in body weights of the animals in these two groups indicate that long-term exposure at these levels of DSP-Visulex dosing (i.e., 15 and 25% DSP for 20 minutes) may have significant systemic side effects on rabbit. Since all animals exhibited systemic exposure of both DSP and DEX after single administration of the DSP-Visulex (discussed above), this is an expected outcome after multiple treatments of DSP-Visulex for 3 months [42, 43]. It should be noted that the 20-minute treatment duration and 25% DSP tested in this study were an exaggerated wearing time and concentration to find the adverse effect (if any). The intended clinical use in the patient population would be 10 minutes or less and the DSP concentration would be 15% or less.

In summary, repeated 20-minute weekly treatments of 4 and 8% DSP-Visulex are well tolerated over 3 months, whereas, respective 15 and 25% DSP-Visulex treatments potentially are limited to shorter periods of time, perhaps between 4 and 8 weeks. The safety of DSP-Visulex with a shorter application time (i.e., 8 and 15% DSP for 5 minutes) was evaluated in phase I/II clinical trial for the treatment of noninfectious anterior uveitis discussed in a later section.

## 8. Efficacy of DSP-Visulex on an experimental uveitis rabbit model

Experimental uveitis, also known as experimental autoimmune uveitis (EAU), has been a method for evaluation of various therapeutic agents as well as new drug delivery systems for intermediate, posterior, and panuveitis [44–50]. By preimmunization and challenge of Mycobacterium tuberculosis H37Ra antigen, this induction causes a severe panuveitis in rabbit that lasts for more than 4 weeks [44–51].

Single application and multiple applications of DSP-Visulex (i.e., 8 and 15%) have been shown to be effective in treating the experimental uveitis over the course of a 29-day study [34]. In the study, rabbits were randomly assigned into six groups after uveitis induction. Rabbit eyes were examined by indirect ophthalmoscopy. A modified McDonald-Shadduck scale [52] was used for scoring inflammation. An average of all scores over the course of study is calculated for comparison. The eyes were collected at the end of the study on Day 29 for histopathology evaluation.

All induced eyes showed signs of inflammation within a day after the uveitic induction. Overall, inflammation occurred more significantly in the posterior chamber than in the anterior chamber (**Tables 3** and **4**). The most apparent finding from the eye examination in assessing the severity of uveitis is inflammation in vitreous (**Figure 4** and **Table 3**). All animals in the control group (untreated) reached a severe vitritis, which remained on average above a score of 3 through the end of study. The average inflammation score of vitreous for the control group was significantly higher than all the DSP-Visulex treatment groups. The resolution speed of inflammation in the vitreous appears

| Treatment Regimen | Inflammation Score | | |
|---|---|---|---|
| | Conjunctival injection | Anterior Chamber | Vitreous |
| Group 1: Control (No treatment) | 0.9 ± 0.8 | 0.5 ± 0.5 | 3.3 ± 1.1 |
| Group 2: 15% DSP (15min, 4 doses) | 0.5 ± 0.4** | 0.1 ± 0.2*** | 0.4 ± 1.0*** |
| Group 3: 15% DSP (10min, 1 dose) | 0.3 ± 0.4*** | 0.1 ± 0.2*** | 0.6 ± 1.2*** |
| Group 4: 8% DSP (10min, 1 dose) | 0.5 ± 0.5** | 0.3 ± 0.4** | 0.4 ± 0.8*** |
| Group 5: 8% DSP (5 min, 4 doses) | 0.9 ± 0.8 | 0.5 ± 0.5 | 1.4 ± 1.7*** |
| Group 6: 4% DSP (10min, 2 doses) | 0.5 ± 0.5* | 0.4 ± 0.6 | 1.4 ± 1.6*** |

*$^{*}P < .05$, $^{**}P < .01$, and $^{***}P < .001$.*

**Table 3.**
*Inflammation scores from observations using indirect ophthalmoscope.*

to correlate with both the DSP concentration and frequency of DSP-Visulex treatment. The same correlation also corresponds to the inflammation score observed by histopathology (**Table 4**). A complete resolution of the highest dosing regimen was observed at Day 10 and the lowest dosing regimen was observed at Day 22.

Statistical differences in the average scores observed between the control group and each DSP-Visulex treatment group were assessed by the Wilcoxon rank-sum test with $^{*}P < .05$, $^{**}P < .01$, and $^{***}P < .001$.

The signs of inflammation in the anterior section including the anterior chamber (AC) and conjunctiva were mild even with the control group. This made it difficult to see significant differences between the control and the low dosing regimens through the observations using indirect ophthalmoscope. The efficacy of the low dosing regimens for the anterior section was mainly supported by histopathology evaluation (**Table 4**).

For histopathology evaluation, the average inflammation scores for both anterior and posterior sections are presented in **Table 4**. The total inflammatory scores of anterior section were high for the untreated eye; whereas for the DSP-Visulex treatment groups, they were significantly lower. The efficacy of DSP-Visulex treatment in the anterior section appears to be related to DSP concentrations. The

| Treatment Regimen | Total Inflammatory Score of Anterior Section | Inflammatory Cell Infiltration Score | |
|---|---|---|---|
| | | Anterior Section | Posterior Section |
| Group 1: Control (No treatment) | 4.4 ± 2.6 | 0.7 ± 1.0 | 2.9 ± 1.2 |
| Group 2: 15% DSP (15min, 4 doses) | 0.2 ± 0.4*** | 0.0 ± 0.2*** | 0.1 ± 0.3*** |
| Group 3: 15% DSP (10min, 1 dose) | 1.0 ± 1.1** | 0.2 ± 0.4** | 1.8 ± 1.5** |
| Group 4: 8% DSP (10min, 1 dose) | 1.8 ± 0.7** | 0.3 ± 0.7** | 1.2 ± 0.9*** |
| Group 5: 8% DSP (5 min, 4 doses) | 1.4 ± 1.7** | 0.2 ± 0.8*** | 1.9 ± 1.6** |
| Group 6: 4% DSP (10min, 2 doses) | 1.9 ± 1.1* | 0.3 ± 0.7** | 2.9 ± 1.0 |

*$^{*}P < .05$, $^{**}P < .01$, and $^{***}P < .001$.*

**Table 4.**
*Inflammation scores and inflammatory cell infiltration score from histopathology examination*

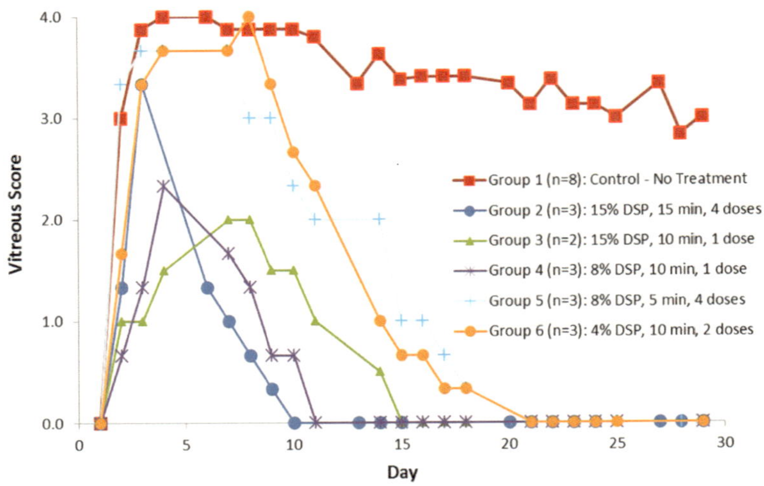


**Figure 4.**
*Vitreous scores of various treatment groups tested in the experimental uveitis rabbit model.*

intermediate and posterior uveitis was persistent in the control group for 29 days, consistent with the ophthalmoscopic observations. The eyes from the highest dose regimen had almost no pathological signs of uveitis present and their posterior tissues appeared to be healthy with minimal inflammation while the untreated eyes appeared to be completely impaired (**Figure 5**). The overall inflammation scores of the posterior section suggest that all DSP-Visulex treatment regimens, except the lowest dosing regimen, were less inflamed in the posterior section than the controls.

The successful treatment with a single-dose of DSP-Visulex was not anticipated in this uveitis model because the DSP was estimated to be cleared from the eye tissues and eventually from the body within 24 hours based on the pharmacokinetics of dexamethasone sodium phosphate [38, 39]. Although the duration of action for dexamethasone can last up to 72 hours [53], it cannot explain the long anti-inflammatory effect of the single dose of DSP-Visulex in this chronic uveitis model, unless a very high dose of DSP (similar to the 8 and 15% DSP-Visulex) can stop the inflammatory process in the uveitic eye without a repeat dose. More studies (e.g., a dose-ranging study of DSP IVT injection in experimental uveitis rabbit) need to be done to confirm this hypothesis.

The uveitis model used in this DSP-Visulex study was similar to (if not the same as) the uveitis rabbit model used in the preclinical studies of intravitreal DEX implant [44, 46]. Considering a qualitative (DEX vs. DSP) and indirect comparison

(A) 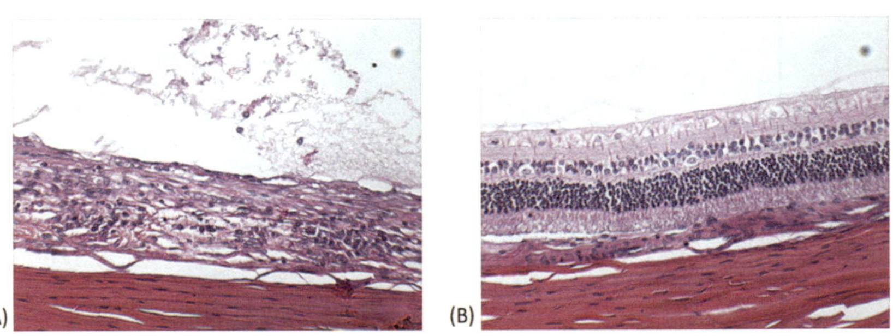 (B)

**Figure 5.**
*Comparative histopathologic presentation of the posterior section of the eyes at the end of study (Day 29). (A) Control (untreated eye): The inflammation is severe and the photoreceptor layer is completely damaged. (B) 15% DSP (15 minutes, 4 doses): Inflammation is minimal and the tissue structure is well preserved.*

(nonhuman primate vs. rabbit) to intravitreal DEX implant (Ozurdex®) from a pharmacokinetic study in nonhuman primate [41], the $C_{max}$ of DEX from Ozurdex® was 1.1 μg/g in the retina at Day 60 and 0.2 μg/mL in the vitreous at Day 60 whereas the concentration of DSP in the retina-choroid and vitreous from DSP-Visulex was much higher immediately after a single administration (i.e., ≥18 μg/g in the retina-choroid and ≥ 1 μg/mL in vitreous) [35]. This may suggest a more rapid onset of the pharmacological action with DSP-Visulex compared to Ozurdex®. However, since Ozurdex®, which is a controlled release product, provides a much longer exposure of DEX in eyes compared to DSP-Visulex, the risks and benefits of the two products in the eye diseases will need to be further evaluated, particularly in well-controlled efficacy models.

In summary, the ophthalmoscopic observations and histopathological examinations strongly indicate that the DSP-Visulex treatment was safe and well tolerated in the rabbit uveitis model. Overall, all the 8 and 15% DSP-Visulex treatment regimens in this study can be considered for the treatment of anterior, intermediate, posterior, and panuveitis. On the other hand, the 4% DSP-Visulex regimen may only be considered for the treatment of anterior and intermediate uveitis but not for posterior uveitis unless more frequent dosing is tested.

## 9. Safety and efficacy of DSP-Visulex for noninfectious anterior uveitis: a randomized phase I/II clinical trial

DSP-Visulex treatment regimens (two applications on the first week and then weekly after) were evaluated for safety and efficacy against daily prednisolone acetate eye drop (PA) for noninfectious anterior uveitis[54]. The study (called DSPV-201) was a phase I/II, multicenter, randomized, parallel group, double-masked, active-controlled, and dose comparison study.

A total of 44 patients were randomized in 1:1:1 ratio to the three treatment groups: 14 patients to the 8% group (8% DSP-Visulex with placebo eye drops), 15 patients to the 15% group (15% DSP-Visulex with placebo eye drops), and 15 patients to the PA group (Vehicle-Visulex with 1% PA eye drops). All patients received the Visulex treatments (either DSP-Visulex or Vehicle-Visulex) at Visit 1 (Day 1), Visit 2 (Day 3 ± 1), Visit 3 (Day 8 ± 1), and Visit 4 (Day 15 ± 1) with an optional Visulex treatment at Visit 5 (Day 22 ± 1). The optional Visulex treatment was at the investigator's discretion. Patients self-administered the study eye drops 6 times daily through Visit 4, then tapered off. Both safety and efficacy assessments were made at all visits. Efficacy parameters included anterior chamber cell (ACC) count and anterior chamber flare (ACF) grade, which were graded based on the Standardization of Uveitis Nomenclature (SUN) Working Group classification [55]. The safety parameters assessed were the incidence of treatment-emergent adverse events (AEs), best-corrected visual acuity (BCVA), intraocular pressure (IOP), slit lamp biomicroscopy assessments, ophthalmoscopy assessments, and ocular pain.

A total of 40 patients completed the study: 12 patients in the 8% group, 14 patients in the 15% group, and 14 patients in the PA group. The patient characteristics regarding age, gender, and race were comparable among the three groups [54]. The uveitis baseline of the three treatment groups including anterior chamber cell (ACC) grade, anterior chamber flare (ACF) grade, VAS for pain, visual acuity, and IOP were similar. Moreover, the baseline characteristics were also comparable to larger phase III studies [54, 56].

The percentages of patients with zero ACC count were comparable among all three treatment groups at the end of the study (**Figure 6A**). The profiles of ACC clearing over the course of the study are similar among the three treatment groups

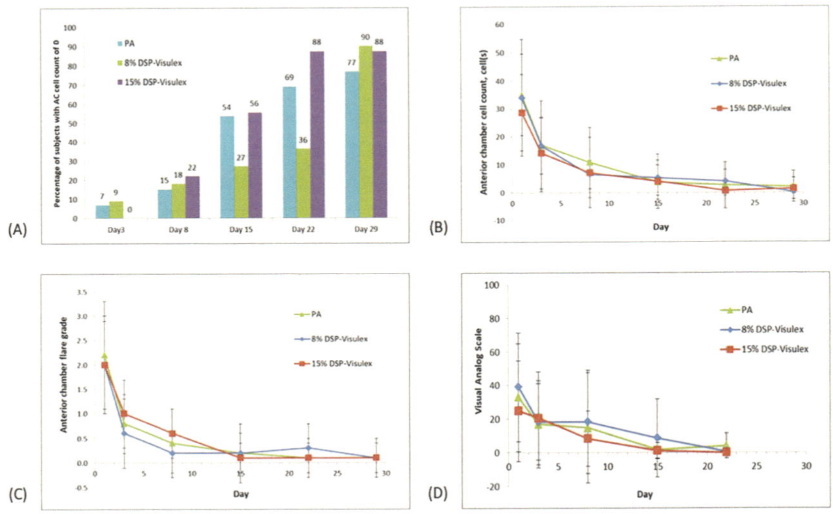


**Figure 6.**
*(A) Percentage of patients with anterior chamber cell count of 0. (B) Anterior chamber cell count. (C) Anterior chamber flare grade based on SUN classification. (D) Ocular pain measured by a visual analog scale.*

(**Figure 6B**). All showed a rapid reduction of ACC counts to the average of 5 cells or lower within 14 days, then gradually approaching 0 cell subsequently. The same trends were also observed with respect to ACF. The 15% illustrated a trend for stronger potency compared with the 8% on the basis of the percent of patients with ACC count of 0 at Visit 5 (Day 22) and the need for an optional dose at Visit 5. Based on the criteria of the SUN working group on the short-term evaluation of a new therapy (i.e., a two-grade decrease in ACC grade or decrease to grade 0 is considered sufficient improvements) [55], weekly DSP-Visulex treatments are considered effective therapy for noninfectious anterior uveitis. Majority of patients in all groups showed similar improvement in visual acuity (i.e., the reductions of logMAR) [54].

The eye pain was measured by visual analog scale (VAS). The reduction in VAS pain scores throughout the study (**Figure 6D**), which coincided with the improvement of other aspects of anterior uveitis, including ACC and ACF, demonstrated that while patients had moderate pain at enrollment, the patients experienced minimal or no pain by the conclusion of the study. These observations can be attributable to either an improvement in symptoms related to a treatment effect of the anterior segment inflammation and/or acquired tolerance to the treatment modality itself over time, the differential effects being difficult to clearly delineate.

No safety concerns were identified in the study. Overall, 19 of 44 patients reported 58 AEs, of which 54 were ocular. The numbers of AE reports from each group were 10, 36, and 12 for the 8%, 15%, and PA groups, respectively. A summary of AEs is presented in **Table 5**. The higher ocular AEs reported with the 15% group are possibly due to the hypertonicity of the 15% DSP formulation compared with the isotonic formulations of 8% DSP and 1% prednisolone acetate, resulting in more ocular irritation. Most AEs were related to ocular surface phenomena. The most frequently reported AEs were corneal abrasion (n = 4), conjunctival staining (n = 4), and cornea staining (n = 4). These findings are consistent with preclinical studies [35] and such AEs are similar to those found with contact lens wearers [57–59]. The AEs are believed to be caused by physical/mechanical abrasion of the Visulex applicator on the corneal and conjunctival surface (i.e., epithelium). Two patients experienced a serious adverse event (SAE), including hospitalization for diabetic ketoacidosis and surgical treatment for unilateral retinal detachment. Both of these SAEs were identified as unrelated to the investigational product. Throughout the

| | 8%DSP-Visulex (N=14) | 15%DSP-Visulex (N=15) | Prednisolone Acetate (N=15) |
|---|---|---|---|
| **General** | | | |
| Patients reporting Any AEs | 7 | 9 | 3 |
| - Suspected drug-related AE | 2 | 6 | 2 |
| - Not suspected drug-related AE | 5 | 3 | 1 |
| **Treatment-emergent AEs** | | | |
| Conjunctival haemorrhage | 1 | 0 | 0 |
| Conjunctival edema | 0 | 0 | 1 |
| Eye pain | 0 | 1 | 2 |
| Eyelid pain | 0 | 1 | 0 |
| Glaucoma | 0 | 1 | 0 |
| Keratic precipitates | 0 | 1 | 0 |
| Keratitis | 0 | 1 | 0 |
| Ocular hyperemia | 0 | 1 | 0 |
| Retinal detachment | 1 | 0 | 0 |
| Retinal haemorrhage | 1 | 0 | 0 |
| Uveitis | 0 | 2 | 0 |
| Visual acuity reduced | 0 | 1 | 0 |
| Conjunctivitis | 0 | 1 | 0 |
| Conjunctivitis viral | 1 | 0 | 0 |
| Gastroenteritis viral | 0 | 1 | 0 |
| Nasopharyngitis | 1 | 0 | 0 |
| Corneal abrasion | 1 | 3 | 0 |
| Conjunctival staining | 1 | 2 | 1 |
| Vital dye staining cornea present | 1 | 2 | 1 |
| Diabetic ketoacidosis | 0 | 0 | 1 |
| Headache | 0 | 0 | 1 |
| Granulomatous dermatitis | 1 | 0 | 0 |

**Table 5.**
*Adverse events.*

course of this study, no apparent corticosteroid-mediated AEs were observed and only four reported AEs were even considered as systemic AEs (three were from PA group and one, which was granulomatous dermatitis, was from the 8% group). None of the systemic AEs were considered treatment-related. These findings suggest negligible systemic exposure of DSP-Visulex in human as discussed above. The safety outcomes of PA are consistent with expectations and the incidence of AEs are comparable to other clinical studies [56, 60]. This suggests that the Visulex applicator by itself contributes minimally to any adverse effects and tolerability.

The results of IOP elevation in the PA arm (**Figure** 7) are consistent with a phase 3 study of PA in treating noninfectious anterior uveitis [56] and other local corticosteroid treatments including eye drops, intravitreal injection, periocular injections, and intravitreal implants [61]. With respect to the DSP-Visulex arms, no IOP elevation was observed after the first week of treatment. The IOP results from both DSP-Visulex groups are not congruent with those typically observed for topical steroid treatments. However, this outcome is consistent with the preclinical studies of DSP-Visulex in rabbits, in which IOP elevations are minimal and transient (unpublished data). We hypothesize that the length of steroid exposure to the eye, which is the main difference between the DSP-Visulex treatment and the other corticosteroid therapies,

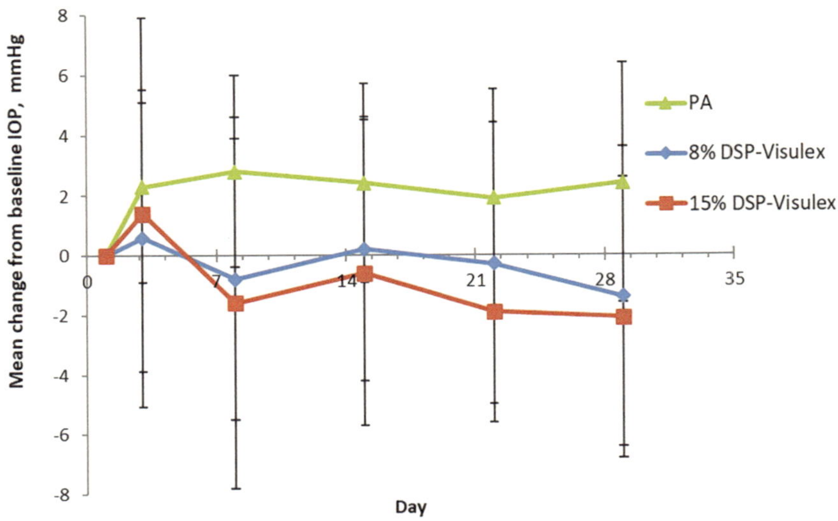


**Figure 7.**
*Mean changes in intraocular pressure (IOP) from baseline.*

affects the IOP elevation. Frequent daily eye drops, sustained release implants, and IVT injections of corticosteroid suspensions represent constant drug exposure to eye tissues including trabecular meshwork. By contrast, the steroid exposure to the eye in the case of DSP-Visulex is intermittent (i.e., twice in the first week and then once a week thereafter). We speculate that this unique pulsatile treatment of DSP-Visulex optimizes the balance between the anti-inflammatory and IOP effects of steroid therapy. Furthermore, the delivery method of steroid into the AC with DSP-Visulex may be analogous to that of a micropulse of relatively high concentration of local steroid into the eye, and that frequent micropulse of steroid may be more efficacious from inflammatory perspective and not over expose trabecular meshwork to more sustained concentrations of steroid over a long period of time. Glaucoma, diabetic, or elderly patients who are more susceptible to the IOP increases could benefit from DSP-Visulex treatments. However, this plausible benefit of IOP along with the efficacy and safety must be confirmed in a pivotal study with a larger sample size.

## 10. DSP-Visulex compared to an iontophoresis of dexamethasone phosphate

It is of interest to compare two novel ocular drug delivery systems of dexamethasone phosphate: one employs electrical current (also known as iontophoresis) and another is based on passive diffusion (i.e., no electrical current). On a semi-quantitative basis, the present DSP-Visulex results may be compared to the ocular iontophoresis results of 4% dexamethasone phosphate as reported by Güngör et al.[62]. The 8% DSP-Visulex (5-minute application or longer) appears to deliver DSP to retina-choroid tissues to the same extent as the iontophoresis results (5-minute application at 2, 4, and 6 mA) and the 15 and 25% DSP-Visulex appear to be somewhat better than the iontophoresis results.

An iontophoresis of dexamethasone phosphate, known as EGP-437, is also being investigated in clinical studies for noninfectious anterior uveitis. While not directly comparable, in the phase 2 clinical trial of EGP-437 for noninfectious anterior uveitis [40], the percentage of patients achieving the ACC score of zero were

48% at Day 14 and 60% at Day 28 for EGP-437, whereas, the respective percentage of DSP-Visulex patients in the present study achieving the ACC score of zero were approximately 41% at Day 15 and 89% at Day 29. In the phase 2 study of EGP-437, it appeared that the higher the electrical current used, the lesser the efficacy. While this was an unexpected outcome of the EGP-437 study, Pescina et al. [63] suggested that under certain iontophoretic conditions used in the study of EGP-437, the electroosmotic flow occurring during iontophoresis may oppose the direction of drug transport into ocular tissues resulting in an inverse relationship of electrical current and efficacy. As for safety comparisons, the number of ocular AEs produced from a single dose of EGP-437 is higher than those following multiple applications of DSP-Visulex. Although the comparative discussions of the two studies are qualitative, the results of the DSP-Visulex study may raise a question of the fundamental utility of iontophoresis in DSP administration for the treatment of noninfectious anterior uveitis.

## 11. Conclusion

DSP-Visulex may address problems of existing corticosteroid treatments for uveitis and other eye diseases. This includes eliminating the need for frequent dosing of eye drops (i.e., multiple drops 6–10 times/day), reducing side effects inherent with systemic drug therapies, and avoiding serious risks associated with intravitreal and periocular injections. Data suggest that DSP-Visulex has clinical potential for the noninvasive treatment of ocular diseases including uveitis, macular edema, postoperative inflammation, diabetic retinopathy, and age-related macular degeneration. In the future, many other drug molecules can be incorporated into the Visulex-P platform for various ophthalmic applications. With the positive outcomes of DSP and other in-house-tested therapeutic molecules (e.g., mycophenolic acid, rapamycin, triamcinolone acetonide phosphate, and lipoic acid), we are optimistic that Visulex-P is a new ophthalmic drug delivery system that can benefit both anterior and posterior eye diseases.

## Acknowledgements

The research and development of DSP-Visulex were financially supported by NEI SBIR Grant R44EY014772 and Aciont Inc. The authors thank Dr. Kevin Li at University of Cincinnati for his comments on an early draft, Dr. Nick Mamalis and Dr. Albert Vitale at Moran for their medical insights and helpful discussion on uveitis, Dr. David Miller at Keystone Pharmacy for his help on the study supplies, Dr. Gregory DeNaeyer for his insights on ocular lens design, and Aciont research team for their contributions to this project. This chapter is derived in part from three articles published in: Current Eye Research available online https://doi.org/10.1080/02713683.2018.1540707, Journal of Ocular Pharmacology and Therapeutics available online https://doi.org/10.1089/jop.2017.0093, and https://doi.org/10.1089/jop.2017.0053.

## Conflict of interest

Kongnara Papangkorn, and John Higuchi are employees of Aciont, Inc. Balbir Brar is a consultant at Aciont, Inc. William Higuchi is a founder and CTO of Aciont, Inc.

## Author details

Kongnara Papangkorn*, John W. Higuchi, Balbir Brar and William I. Higuchi
Aciont Inc., Salt Lake City, UT, United States

*Address all correspondence to: kpapangkorn@aciont.com

## References

[1] Nussenblatt RB. The natural history of uveitis. International Ophthalmology. 1990;**14**:303-308

[2] Tomkins-Netzer O, Talat L, Bar A, et al. Long-term clinical outcome and causes of vision loss in patients with uveitis. Ophthalmology. 2014;**121**:2387-2392

[3] Gritz DC, Schwaber EJ, Wong IG. Complications of Uveitis: The Northern California Epidemiology of Uveitis Study. Ocular Immunology and Inflammation. 2017:1-11

[4] Gritz DC, Wong IG. Incidence and prevalence of uveitis in Northern California: The Northern California Epidemiology of Uveitis Study. Ophthalmology. 2004;**111**:491-500

[5] Acharya NR, Tham VM, Esterberg E, et al. Incidence and prevalence of uveitis: Results from the Pacific Ocular Inflammation Study. JAMA Ophthalmology. 2013;**131**:1405-1412

[6] Suhler EB, Lloyd MJ, Choi D, et al. Incidence and Prevalence of Uveitis in Veterans Affairs Medical Centers of the Pacific Northwest. American Journal of Ophthalmology. 2008;**146**:890

[7] Rothova A. Corticosteroids in uveitis. Ophthalmology Clinics of North America. 2002;**15**:389-394

[8] Rohdewald P, Mollmann H, Barth J, et al. Pharmacokinetics of dexamethasone and its phosphate ester. Biopharmaceutics & Drug Disposition. 1987;**8**:205-212

[9] Lee VHL. Esterase activities in adult rabbit eyes. Journal of Pharmaceutical Sciences. 1983;**72**:239-244

[10] Rodriguez Villanueva J, Rodriguez Villanueva L, Guzman Navarro M. Pharmaceutical technology can turn a traditional drug, dexamethasone into a first-line ocular medicine. A global perspective and future trends. International Journal of Pharmaceutics. 2017;**516**:342-351

[11] Urtti A. Challenges and obstacles of ocular pharmacokinetics and drug delivery. Advanced Drug Delivery Reviews. 2006;**58**:1131-1135

[12] Foster CS, Kothari S, Anesi SD, et al. The Ocular Immunology and Uveitis Foundation preferred practice patterns of uveitis management. Survey of Ophthalmology. 2016;**61**:1-17

[13] Yellepeddi VK, Palakurthi S. Recent advances in topical ocular drug delivery. Journal of Ocular Pharmacology and Therapeutics. 2016;**32**:67-82

[14] Novack GD, Robin AL. Ocular pharmacology. Journal of Clinical Pharmacology. 2016;**56**:517-527

[15] Jager RD, Aiello LP, Patel SC, et al. Risks of intravitreous injection: A comprehensive review. Retina. 2004;**24**:676-698

[16] Sen HN, Vitale S, Gangaputra SS, et al. Periocular corticosteroid injections in uveitis: Effects and complications. Ophthalmology. 2014;**121**:2275-2286

[17] Geck U, Pustolla N, Baraki H, et al. Posterior vitreous detachment following intravitreal drug injection. Graefe's Archive for Clinical and Experimental Ophthalmology. 2013;**251**:1691-1695

[18] Lowder C, Belfort R, Lightman S, et al. Dexamethasone intravitreal implant for noninfectious intermediate or posterior uveitis. Archives of Ophthalmology. 2011;**129**:545-553

[19] Boddu SH, Gupta H, Patel S. Drug delivery to the back of the eye following

topical administration: An update on research and patenting activity. Recent Patents on Drug Delivery & Formulation. 2014;**8**:27-36

[20] Hughes PM, Olejnik O, Chang-Lin JE, et al. Topical and systemic drug delivery to the posterior segments. Advanced Drug Delivery Reviews. 2005;**57**:2010-2032

[21] Koevary SB. Pharmacokinetics of topical ocular drug delivery: Potential uses for the treatment of diseases of the posterior segment and beyond. Current Drug Metabolism. 2003;**4**:213-222

[22] Loftsson T, Sigurdsson HH, Konrádsdóttir F, et al. Topical drug delivery to the posterior segment of the eye: Anatomical and physiological considerations. Pharmazie. 2008;**63**:171-179

[23] Ying L, Tahara K, Takeuchi H. Drug delivery to the ocular posterior segment using lipid emulsion via eye drop administration: Effect of emulsion formulations and surface modification. International Journal of Pharmaceutics. 2013;**453**:329-335

[24] Patel A, Cholkar K, Agrahari V, et al. Ocular drug delivery systems: An overview. World Journal Pharmacology. 2013;**2**:47-64

[25] Sigurdsson HH, Konrádsdóttir F, Loftsson T, et al. Topical and systemic absorption in delivery of dexamethasone to the anterior and posterior segments of the eye. Acta Ophthalmologica Scandinavica. 2007;**85**:598-602

[26] Tanito M, Hara K, Takai Y, et al. Topical dexamethasone-cyclodextrin microparticle eye drops for diabetic macular edema. Investigative Ophthalmology and Visual Science. 2011;**52**:7944-7948

[27] Ohira A, Hara K, Jóhannesson G, et al. Topical dexamethasone γ-cyclodextrin nanoparticle eye drops increase visual acuity and decrease macular thickness in diabetic macular oedema. Acta Ophthalmologica. 2015;**93**:610-615

[28] Shulman S, Johannesson G, Stefansson E, et al. Topical dexamethasone-cyclodextrin nanoparticle eye drops for non-infectious Uveitic macular oedema and vitritis: A pilot study. Acta Ophthalmologica. 2015;**93**:411-415

[29] Shikamura Y, Ohtori A, Tojo K. Drug penetration of the posterior eye tissues after topical instillation: In vivo and in silico simulation. Chemical & Pharmaceutical Bulletin (Tokyo). 2011;**59**:1263-1267

[30] Geroski DH, Edelhauser HF. Transscleral drug delivery for posterior segment disease. Advanced Drug Delivery Reviews. 2001;**52**:37-48

[31] Gaudana R, Ananthula HK, Parenky A, et al. Ocular drug delivery. The AAPS Journal. 2010;**12**:348-360

[32] Berezovsky DE, Patel SR, McCarey BE, et al. In vivo ocular fluorophotometry: Delivery of fluoresceinated dextrans via transscleral diffusion in rabbits. Investigative Ophthalmology and Visual Science. 2011;**52**:7038-7045

[33] Miller DJ, Li SK, Tuitupou AL, et al. Passive and oxymetazoline-enhanced delivery with a lens device: Pharmacokinetics and efficacy studies with rabbits. Journal of Ocular Pharmacology and Therapeutics. 2008;**24**:385-391

[34] Papangkorn K, Prendergast E, Higuchi JW, et al. Noninvasive ocular drug delivery system of dexamethasone sodium phosphate in the treatment of experimental uveitis rabbit. Journal of Ocular Pharmacology and Therapeutics. 2017;**33**:753-762

[35] Papangkorn K, Higuchi JW, Brar B, et al. Ocular drug distribution and safety of a noninvasive ocular drug delivery system of dexamethasone sodium phosphate in rabbit. Journal of Ocular Pharmacology and Therapeutics. 2018;**34**:325-334

[36] Weijtens O, Schoemaker RC, Lentjes EGWM, et al. Dexamethasone concentration in the subretinal fluid after a subconjunctival injection, a peribulbar injection, or an oral dose. Ophthalmology. 2000;**107**:1932-1938

[37] Weijtens O, Schoemaker RC, Romijn FPHTM, et al. Intraocular penetration and systemic absorption after topical application of dexamethasone disodium phosphate. Ophthalmology. 2002;**109**:1887-1891

[38] Hosseini K, Matsushima D, Johnson J, et al. Pharmacokinetic study of dexamethasone disodium phosphate using intravitreal, subconjunctival, and intravenous delivery routes in rabbits. Journal of Ocular Pharmacology and Therapeutics. 2008;**24**:301-308

[39] Czock D, Keller F, Rasche FM, et al. Pharmacokinetics and pharmacodynamics of systemically administered glucocorticoids. Clinical Pharmacokinetics. 2005;**44**:61-98

[40] Cohen AE, Assang C, Patane MA, et al. Evaluation of dexamethasone phosphate delivered by ocular iontophoresis for treating noninfectious anterior uveitis. Ophthalmology. 2012;**119**:66-73

[41] Chang-Lin J-E, Attar M, Acheampong AA, et al. Pharmacokinetics and pharmacodynamics of the sustained-release dexamethasone intravitreal implant. Investigative Ophthalmology & Visual Science. 2010:80-86

[42] Patane MA, Schubert W, Sanford T, et al. Evaluation of ocular and general safety following repeated dosing of dexamethasone phosphate delivered by transscleral iontophoresis in rabbits. Journal of Ocular Pharmacology and Therapeutics. 2013;**29**:760-769

[43] Rosenthal KL. Therapeutic contraindications in exotic pets. Seminars in Avian and Exotic Pet Medicine. 2004;**13**:44-48

[44] Cheng CK, Berger AS, Pearson PA, et al. Intravitreal sustained-release dexamethasone device in the treatment of experimental uveitis. Investigative Ophthalmology and Visual Science. 1995;**36**:442-453

[45] Ang M, Ng X, Wong C, et al. Evaluation of a prednisolone acetate-loaded subconjunctival implant for the treatment of recurrent uveitis in a rabbit model. PLoS One. 2014;**9**:e97555

[46] Ghosn CR, Li Y, Orilla WC, et al. Treatment of experimental anterior and intermediate uveitis by a dexamethasone intravitreal implant. Investigative Ophthalmology and Visual Science. 2011;**52**:2917-2923

[47] Eperon S, Balaskas K, Vaudaux J, et al. Experimental uveitis can be maintained in rabbits for a period of six weeks after a safe sensitization method. Current Eye Research. 2013;**38**:405-412

[48] Jaffe GJ, Yang CS, Wang XC, et al. Intravitreal sustained-release cyclosporine in the treatment of experimental uveitis. Ophthalmology. 1998;**105**:46-56

[49] Sloper CM, Powell RJ, Dua HS. Tacrolimus (FK506) in the treatment of posterior uveitis refractory to cyclosporine. Ophthalmology. 1999;**106**:723-728

[50] Sakurai E, Nozaki M, Okabe K, et al. Scleral Plug of Biodegradable Polymers Containing Tacrolimus (FK506) for Experimental Uveitis.

Investigative Ophthalmology and Visual Science. 2003;**44**:4845-4852

[51] Jubb ÊVF, Kennedy PC, Palmer N. Pathology of Domestic Animals. 4th ed. San Diago: Academic Press; 1993

[52] Hackett R, McDonald T. Eye irritation. In: Marzulli F, Maibach H, editors. Advances in Modern Toxicology: Dermatoxicology. Washington, DC: Hemisphere Publishing; 1991. pp. 749-815

[53] Schimmer BP, Parker KL. Chapter 60. Adrenocorticotropic hormone; adrenocortical steroids and their synthetic analogs; inhibitors of the synthesis and actions of adrenocortical hormones. In: Goodman & Gilman's The Pharmacological Basis of Therapeutics. 10th ed. McGraw-Hill; 2001

[54] Papangkorn K, Truett KR, Vitale AT, et al. Novel dexamethasone sodium phosphate treatment (DSP-Visulex) for non-infectious anterior uveitis: A randomized phase i/ii clinical trial. Current Eye Research. Epub ahead of print 2018. DOI: 10.1080/02713683.2018.1540707

[55] Jabs DA, Nussenblatt RB, Rosenbaum JT, et al. Standardization of uveitis nomenclature for reporting clinical data. Results of the First International Workshop. American Journal of Ophthalmology. 2005;**140**:509-516

[56] Sheppard JD, Toyos MM, Kempen JH, et al. Difluprednate 0.05% versus prednisolone acetate 1% for endogenous anterior uveitis: A phase III, multicenter, randomized study. Investigative Ophthalmology and Visual Science. 2014;**55**:2993-3002

[57] Nichols KK, Mitchell GL, Simon KM, et al. Corneal staining in hydrogel lens wearers. Optometry and Vision Science. 2002;**79**:20-30

[58] Fonn D, Peterson RC, Woods CA. Corneal staining as a response to contact lens wear. Eye & Contact Lens. 2010;**36**:318-321

[59] Schein OD. Adverse reactions associated with contact lens use. In: Flattau PE, editor. Considerations in Contact Lens Use Under Adverse Conditions: Proceedings of a Symposium. Washington, D.C.: National Academies Press; 1991. pp. 58-67

[60] Foster CS, Davanzo R, Flynn TE, et al. Durezol (Difluprednate Ophthalmic Emulsion 0.05%) compared with Pred Forte 1% ophthalmic suspension in the treatment of endogenous anterior uveitis. Journal of Ocular Pharmacology and Therapeutics. 2010;**26**:475-483

[61] Razeghinejad MR, Katz LJ. Steroid-induced iatrogenic glaucoma. Ophthalmic Research. 2012;**47**:66-80

[62] Güngör S, Delgado-Charro MB, Ruiz-Perez B, et al. Trans-scleral iontophoretic delivery of low molecular weight therapeutics. Journal of Controlled Release. 2010;**147**:225-231

[63] Pescina S, Martini D, Santi P, et al. In vitro trans-scleral iontophoresis of methylprednisolone hemisuccinate with short application time and high drug concentration. International Journal of Pharmaceutics. 2013;**451**:12-17

Chapter 7

# Biological Therapies that Target Inflammatory Cytokines to Treat Uveitis

*Ashvini Reddy, Fauziyya Muhammad and Darren J. Lee*

## Abstract

Uveitis is a leading cause of blindness that presents a considerable challenge given that our understanding of the mechanisms of disease is still evolving. Both innate and adaptive immunity play a role in disease and mediators of these responses can serve as therapeutic targets. TNF-α and IL-1β inflammatory cytokines are central mediators of immunity and are involved in the dysregulated inflammatory response during uveitis. Because toxicity limits the use of steroids and other steroid-sparing agents, biologics that target a specific cell type or pathway are being explored for the treatment of autoimmune uveitis. This chapter begins with a broad overview of the aberrant immune response resulting in uveitis, and highlights key mediators such as TNF-α, IL-1β, IL-6, and IL-17 and their potential use as therapeutic targets. Most biological agents discussed in this review have not been FDA-approved for uveitis. However, favorable outcomes in early trials and FDA approval of these drugs for the treatment of other autoimmune diseases associated with uveitis support the potential for these biological agents in the management of uveitis. This review aims to provide an updated report on the efficacy of biologics that target TNF-α, IL-1β, IL-6, and IL-17 for the treatment of autoimmune uveitis.

**Keywords:** uveitis, TNF-α, IL-1β, IL-6, IL-17, etanercept, adalimumab, infliximab, golimumab, certolizumab, anakinra, canakinumab, gevokizumab, rilonacept, tocilizumab, sarilumab, secukinumab

## 1. Introduction

Uveitis is the third leading cause of blindness in western countries and fourth worldwide [1, 2]. The ocular inflammation associated with uveitis can occur in every tissue within the eye so is frequently described according to the anatomical location of the inflammation [3, 4]. Anterior uveitis includes inflammation of the iris, ciliary body, and anterior chamber. Intermediate uveitis involves the vitreous and pars plana, while posterior uveitis describes inflammation of the retina and choroid [5, 6]. Sometimes, both anterior or intermediate and posterior uveitides can occur, which is referred to as panuveitis [5, 6]. Uveitis can be due to infectious or noninfectious causes; the latter is thought to be immune mediated and is commonly referred to as autoimmune uveitis (AU) [7, 8]. Both infectious and noninfectious uveitides lead to damaging inflammation, and undertreatment leads to destruction of ocular tissue which can result in vision loss [9, 10]. So, the goal of treatment is to suppress the ocular inflammation to preserve vision [7]. Generally, uveitis of infectious origin is treated with systemic and/or local antibiotics, antivirals, or antifungals, and inflammation usually resolves once the pathogen is eliminated [7]. Because noninfectious uveitis is immune-mediated, suppression of the immune system is necessary [7, 11].

The current treatment paradigm for noninfectious uveitis is to treat with medications that suppress the immune system to drive the inflammatory response into remission [2, 7]. Corticosteroids can be given locally and/or systemically to rapidly suppress inflammation, but they are not a long-term treatment option due to their side effects [7, 12–14]. When the steroids are discontinued, there is a risk of recurrent disease [15]. Localized slow-releasing steroid implants have been developed and have shown some efficacy, but these can result in cataract and glaucoma [14, 16]. As such, immunomodulating or immunosuppressants are used concomitantly to supplement or taper off the steroids in severe or chronic cases [7]. These immunosuppressive therapies, also called "steroid-sparing drugs," include nonsteroidal anti-inflammatory drugs (NSAIDs); antimetabolites such as methotrexate, azathioprine, and mycophenolate; T-cell inhibitors such as tacrolimus; and cyclosporine and mTOR inhibitors such as rapamycin and derivatives of rapamycin [2, 7]. Also, DNA alkylating agents such as chlorambucil and cyclophosphamide can also be utilized. The steroid-sparing drugs have significantly improved the outcome of uveitis and provide additional more targeted treatment options [17]. However, as with steroids, these drugs may produce significant side effects, including an increased susceptibility to infection, and many still fail to provide lasting remission [2, 18]. It is conceivable that a targeted therapy that only suppresses one or two inflammatory pathways may offer a more favorable side effect profile than standard steroid-sparing agents [2]. Biologics are a relatively new class of medications that specifically target specific molecules involved in inflammation. The major hurdles to implement biological therapies include a large financial burden and questions about long-term efficacy. Therefore, in this report we discuss the outcomes of treating uveitis with biologics with a specific focus on inhibition of TNF-α, IL-1β, IL-6, and IL-17 inflammatory cytokines.

### 1.1 Biologics in uveitis

Progress in the field of ocular immunology has provided a basic understanding of the inflammatory mechanisms that contribute to the pathogenesis of noninfectious uveitis. This allows for a better understanding of the mechanism of action of many medications. Many of the current immunosuppressive therapies suppress inflammation via broad mechanisms of action. For example, mycophenolate inhibits expansion and survival of lymphocytes by limiting the transport of purines into the cell, thus preventing proliferation of T cells and B cells which are dependent on extracellular purines [19]. The disadvantage of this strategy is that differentiation of regulatory T cells (Tregs), a subset of T cells, that have been demonstrated to suppress autoimmune disease would also be inhibited [20, 21]. Rapamycin inhibition of mTOR is effective in suppressing rapidly dividing cells such as leukocytes, but the mTOR pathway is utilized by many cells in the body, so mTOR inhibitors are associated with a wide array of side effects [22]. Therefore, the effective treatment of autoimmune uveitis with a minimal side effect is dependent on the development of much more targeted treatments.

A better understanding of autoimmune diseases and specifically of ocular immunology now provides the possibility of specifically targeting important inflammatory pathways rather than broadly suppressing the immune response [14]. One such method to target specific inflammatory cytokines or receptors is with the use of biologics [2, 14, 23]. The biological agents, also called "biological response modifiers" or "biologics," are a broad group of molecules that have been utilized to interfere and alter inflammation during immune-mediated processes [2]. These agents include recombinant cytokines, monoclonal antibodies that target cell surface proteins and receptors, specific antagonists of cytokines, and soluble receptors [14, 24]. These drugs function by specifically suppressing a single pathway through targeting of an effector molecule [14, 23]. As such, biological agents are being used as a treatment for refractory uveitis [25, 26]. Unfortunately, biologics are not always an option because of extremely high costs that limit approval for off-label use by insurance. The justification to insurance can be even more challenging because of the limited number of published reports documenting the effectiveness of biologics. As such, it is necessary to demonstrate that current biologics are effective in providing sustained remission. Therefore, the purpose of this review is to provide a summary of the literature of the outcomes and effectiveness of biologics that target the key inflammatory mediators especially TNF-α, IL-1β, IL-6, and IL-17. In addition, in order to provide a better understanding of the immunological function of these biologics, we will also provide a limited discussion of the immunological pathways that are targeted by TNF-α, IL-1β, IL-6, and IL-17.

### 1.2 Basic immunology of uveitis

Immune-mediated or autoimmune uveitis is a group of heterogeneous diseases that can be restricted to the eye, as in pars planitis or birdshot chorioretinopathy. The vast majority of uveitis patients experience localized inflammation. However, ocular inflammation can also be associated with systemic disease, such as in lupus, ankylosing spondylitis, and multiple sclerosis [27]. There are still many unknown aspects of the pathogenesis of autoimmune uveitis, but results from human and animal research supported potential mechanisms. One theory is the molecular mimicry model, in which the manifestation of autoimmune uveitis is thought to result from clearance of a pathogen with an antigen with a similar structure to a self-antigen in the eye [28–30]. However, the initiating antigens have not been isolated nor is it likely to be identified due to antigenic shift that occurs with chronic tissue inflammation [31]. In some cases, there is a genetic component, as evidenced with gene associations mapping to the HLA locus, such as HLA-B27, HLA-A29, and HLA-B51 [32–34]. HLA-B27 is associated with anterior uveitis, reactive/rheumatoid arthritis, and ankylosing spondylitis. HLA-A29 is associated with birdshot chorioretinopathy, and HLA-B51 is associated with Behcet's disease [35–37]. Because there is not 100% penetrance with these HLA alleles, there is likely also an environmental trigger that is required as well. This demonstrates the heterogeneity associated with autoimmune uveitis and illustrates why a single therapy may not be effective for all uveitis patients. Thus, additional research is necessary to further our understanding of this disease.

Innate and adaptive immune cells are intricately connected during a normal immune response and aberrant responses as in autoimmune uveitis [30, 38]. The trigger of immune activation during uveitis is not well understood, but it is speculated that both environmental and genetic predispositions can initiate an inflammatory response that would eventually cause damage to the eye during uveitis [39, 40]. Innate immune cells such as monocytes, macrophages, and dendritic cells generally respond first to these inflammatory cues [41, 42]. These activated innate immune cells secrete proinflammatory cytokines such as TNF-α, IL-6, and IL-1β which serve as mediators of inflammation [34, 38, 43]. The role of innate immunity in the pathogenesis of uveitis is evident in both human and animal studies, where markers of inflammatory monocytes are more abundant in uveitis patients than their healthy controls [44]. Likewise, high levels of these inflammatory cytokines have been shown to be elevated in the ocular fluids of uveitis patients [45]. Also, animal models of uveitis which recapitulate the pathologies seen in human uveitis require adjuvants in the induction of the T-cell-mediated uveitis [46]. These required adjuvants activate the pattern recognition receptors (PRR) on innate immune cells that result in the production of these TNF-α, IL-1β, and IL-6 [34, 38]. As such, inhibition of TNF-α, IL-1β, and IL-6 is effective in reducing the ocular inflammation observed in numerous mouse models of uveitis [47–49]. Activated innate immune cells can act as antigen-presenting cells (APCs) and/or cytokine-secreting cells to provide signals that activate B and T cells [50]. In response to this activation, T cells differentiate into effector cells and largely produce inflammatory mediators such as cytokines that activate and recruit other immune cells that enhance ocular damage [34].

Several studies have highlighted the involvement of mediators and cellular responses that integrate both innate and adaptive immunities in the pathogenesis of uveitis [30, 41]. In this review, TNF-α, IL-17, IL-6, and IL-1β are the mediators of interest. While TNF-α, IL-6, and IL-1β are central mediators of inflammation that lead to activation of both innate and adaptive immunities, IL-17 is produced by a specific effector T cells (Th17 cells) that has a strong association with autoimmunity [51, 52]. Elevated levels of these cytokines are seen in the ocular fluids and plasma of uveitis patients [53–55].

Biological agents that specifically target these immune mediators or T-cell-activating molecules have gained wide recognition as effective therapy for immune-mediated diseases such as rheumatoid arthritis (RA), juvenile idiopathic arthritis (JIA), psoriasis, sarcoidosis, and organ rejection and are therefore being used for the treatment of uveitis [56]. Results from treatment of animal models and biological samples of uveitis patients with antagonists of the inflammatory mediators have demonstrated the involvement of these mediators with autoimmune uveitis [57, 58]. Currently, there are numerous clinical trials that are testing the efficacies of biological agents for the treatment of autoimmune uveitis.

## 2. TNF-α inhibitors

TNF-α inhibitors are biological agents that target tumor necrosis factor alpha (TNF-α) and its receptors. TNF-α was initially studied for its ability to stimulate necrosis of malignant tumors [59, 60]. An immunological role was later discovered as it is also an important inflammatory mediator [59, 60]. TNF-α is a proinflammatory cytokine that is secreted by many immune cells of the innate and adaptive arm of the immune response, including T cells, and macrophages, and nonimmune cells such as keratinocytes [60]. TNF-α binding to one of the two isoforms of its transmembrane receptor (TNFr1 and TNFr2) is the first step in triggering a response [59]. Binding of TNF ligand to its receptor activates downstream signals that lead to a cascade of cellular events that include cellular proliferation, differentiation, apoptosis, survival, and regulation of inflammatory cytokine production [60]. Because these events lead to activation of inflammatory cells, TNF-α is considered a master regulator of inflammation [60, 61]. TNF-α has been implicated in the pathogenesis of autoimmune uveitis and other immune-mediated diseases especially organ-specific diseases [62–64]. High levels of TNF-α have been reported in the aqueous humor and sera of uveitis patients compared to their healthy controls [65]. Also, elevated levels of this cytokine are observed in the animal models of autoimmune uveitis, and inhibition of TNF-α activity results in disease remission in these animal models [47, 66]. Involvement of TNF-α in many autoimmune diseases has made it a therapeutic target [60]. Currently, there are numerous biologics that target TNF-α activity; these include infliximab, etanercept, adalimumab, golimumab, and certolizumab [67]. Biologics that target TNF-α and its interaction with its receptors were developed and approved for the treatment of autoimmune diseases such as RA, psoriasis, sarcoidosis, inflammatory bowel disease, etc. [67]. The efficacy of TNF-α inhibitors in the treatment of these diseases has led to great interest in the use of these biological agents for the treatment of uveitis.

### 2.1 Etanercept

Etanercept is a recombinant fusion protein that contains the extracellular ligand-binding portion of the human TNF receptor (TNFr2) and the Fc portion of human IgG1 [68]. Because the structure of etanercept contains no membrane-bound portion, it is essentially a soluble TNF receptor that binds the free form of all TNF isoforms (TNF-α, TNF-β, and TNF-γ) [68]. Because the soluble form of TNF and membrane-bound TNF have opposing immunological effects, it is of note that etanercept does not bind to the membrane-bound form [69].

For two decades, etanercept has been used to treat rheumatic diseases, and it is FDA approved for the treatment of JIA, RA, ankylosing spondylitis (AS), psoriatic arthritis (PA), and plaque psoriasis (PP) [68, 70]. Effectiveness of etanercept in the treatment of these diseases led to interest in the use of this drug for uveitis. Etanercept has been reported to be a treatment for refractory uveitis in pediatric patients [71]. In the prospective study, beneficial effects of etanercept were observed in at least 63% of the patients after 3 months of treatment [71]. Another prospective study of the efficacy of etanercept in patients with JIA-associated uveitis showed 73% of the patients had an initial response after 3 months of treatment; however, only about half of the responders (39%) remained in remission after 1 year [72]. In addition, several prospective and retrospective studies of etanercept did not show treatment efficacy in uveitis associated with systemic diseases such as JIA [73], sarcoidosis [74], or chronic uveitis [75]. Some studies have shown an increased incidence of uveitis in patients treated with etanercept for ankylosing spondylitis [76–78]. In general, the efficacy of etanercept for uveitis is poor, and several studies have shown that other TNF inhibitors (adalimumab and infliximab) are more effective and preferred for the treatment of uveitis as discussed below [79, 80].

*Administration and dosing*: Enbrel (Immunex, Thousand Oaks, CA) is the brand name for etanercept, and it is typically administered subcutaneously at a dose of 50 mg every 1–2 weeks or 0.8 mg/kg weekly. It was first approved by the FDA in 1998 for the treatment of rheumatic diseases.

*Adverse effects*: Side effects of etanercept can include localized effects such as pain and swelling at the injection site [81]. There are reported cases of an increased risk of fungal infection and TB reactivation [78, 82]. Some reports have shown exacerbation of uveitis or development of uveitis concurrent with etanercept treatment [78, 82]. Other serious side effects include lupus-like disease due to autoantibodies generated against etanercept, exacerbation of the central and peripheral nervous system demyelinating disorders, hematologic, and cardiovascular side effects [81, 83, 84]. Please see full prescribing information for complete list.

*Contraindications*: Sepsis [85]. Tuberculosis reactivation or newly acquired tuberculosis has been reported to have an increased incidence in patients on TNF inhibitors [86, 87]; additional discussion is provided at the end of this section.

### 2.2 Adalimumab

Adalimumab was the first fully human IgG1 monoclonal antibody to be approved by the FDA. It was approved as an antibody against TNF-α following the development of infliximab and etanercept. Adalimumab inhibits TNF-α activity by directly binding TNF-α to prevent it from interacting with TNF receptors [88]. Adalimumab is FDA approved for the treatment of RA, inflammatory bowel disease, PA, JIA, and AS [89]. Several prospective and retrospective studies report the efficacy of adalimumab in the treatment of uveitis. In a prospective VISUAL I and VISUAL II study (2010 to 2015) of 217 and 226 adult patients with active and inactive uveitis, respectively, Sheppard et al. found significant improvement in clinical outcomes in patients treated with adalimumab compared to the placebo group [90]. Also, a prospective study from 2006 to 2011 showed that 17 out of 19 adult patients with refractory uveitis in Behcet's disease achieved clinical improvement [91]. Similar results were observed in another prospective study with 72 adult patients conducted between 2006 and 2012 [92]. This study reported that adalimumab reduced the frequency of uveitis attacks in patients with AS by 72% [92]. Another prospective study with 31 refractory uveitis patients reported 68% of these patients showed resolution of ocular inflammation at 10 weeks of treatment and after 1 year 39% of these patients maintained remission [93]. Similarly, in a retrospective study, the efficacy and safety of adalimumab in Behcet's disease-related uveitis were reported using records of 40 patients treated with adalimumab for up to 12 months [94]. The retrospective chart review showed remission was achieved in 95% of the patients [94]. The use of adalimumab in pediatric patients was reported in a prospective study with 18 young patients (2–19 years) with chronic anterior uveitis; 88% of the patients responded to the therapy [95]. Similar results were reported in another pediatric study including 90 children and adolescents; this study shows responsiveness to adalimumab and lower treatment failure compared to a placebo treatment [96].

In 2014, the executive committee of the American Uveitis Society recommended adalimumab as a first-line treatment for uveitis associated with Behcet's disease when uncontrolled by standard immunomodulatory drugs [24]. Importantly, in 2016, adalimumab became the first and the only drug to be FDA approved for the treatment of intermediate, posterior, and panuveitis [97].

*Administration and dosing*: Adalimumab is sold under the brand name Humira (AbbVie Inc., North Chicago, IL), and Amjevita is a biosimilar (Amgen, Inc., Thousand Oaks, CA), but Amjevita is not available in the USA due to patent issues, and it is typically given subcutaneously every 1–2 weeks at a dose of 40–80 mg or 20 mg if the body weight is less than 30 kg.

*Adverse effects*: In some of the studies mentioned above, adalimumab treatment for uveitis was associated with some severe side effects. These serious side effects include sarcoidosis, anaphylaxis, optic neuritis, Guillain-Barre syndrome, multiple sclerosis, adenoma, and melanoma [83, 91, 98–100]. Please see full prescribing information for complete list.

*Contraindications*: None are listed with the FDA [101]. Tuberculosis reactivation or newly acquired tuberculosis has been reported to have an increased incidence in patients on TNF inhibitors [86, 87]; additional discussion is provided at the end of this section.

### 2.3 Infliximab

Infliximab is a chimeric IgG1 monoclonal antibody that contains the human constant region and murine variable regions, and it binds both membrane-bound and free TNF-α [102]. This drug was initially developed and approved by the FDA in 1998 for the treatment of inflammatory bowel disease; subsequently, this drug was approved for the treatment of RA and other rheumatoid diseases [103, 104]. Clinical trials to assess the efficacy of infliximab as a treatment for uveitis demonstrate that it is a potential treatment option. One prospective study reported a rapid response to infliximab in six adult patients that had uveitis associated with Behcet's disease or sarcoidosis [105]. Similarly, in another prospective study, 9 out of 11 patients with refractory posterior uveitis showed improvement of disease following treatment with infliximab [106]. Efficacy of infliximab in pediatric patients with uveitis has been demonstrated in retrospective studies of JIA patients [107, 108]. All 17 patients in one study showed a rapid and well-tolerated response to infliximab [108]. Also, several studies have demonstrated the effectiveness of infliximab in localized uveitis as well as systemic autoimmune diseases associated with uveitis. One prospective study demonstrated effective suppression of uveitis in 18 out of 23 patients at 10 weeks of treatment initiation, and clinical success was achieved in all patients at week 50 [109].

Numerous clinical trials have compared the efficacy between adalimumab and infliximab in the treatment of noninfectious uveitis; most of these studies concluded that, overall, both anti-TNF-α agents showed equivalent efficacies. In one study, 160 patients with refractory uveitis were treated with either infliximab or adalimumab, 93% of the patients achieved remission after 12 months of treatment, and no significant difference in terms of occurrence of uveitis was seen between the two treatment groups [110]. Also, the expert panel from the American Uveitis Society recommends infliximab or adalimumab as the first-line treatment for uveitis in Behcet's disease [24].

*Administration and dosing*: Infliximab is sold under the brand name Remicade (Janssen Biotech, Horsham, PA) and is typically given intravenously at a dose of 3–5 mg/kg at weeks 0, 2, 6, and subsequently every 8 weeks [24].

*Adverse effects*: The most notable side effect of infliximab in some patients was generation of autoantibody against the non-humanized component of the drug [111]. Other serious side effects include an increased risk of lymphoma, reactivation of TB, and an increased risk of fungal infections [82]. Infliximab may also contribute to the exacerbation of demyelinating diseases and is not preferred in patients with multiple sclerosis [112, 113]. Please see full prescribing information for complete list.

*Contraindications*: Heart failure has been reported with doses greater than 5 mg/kg. Severe hypersensitivity to Remicade or to inactive components of Remicade or to proteins of mouse origin has been reported [114]. Tuberculosis reactivation or newly acquired tuberculosis has been reported to have an increased incidence in patients on TNF inhibitors [86, 87]; additional discussion is provided at the end of this section.

### 2.4 Golimumab

Golimumab is a promising TNF-α inhibitor for the treatment of autoimmune uveitis. It is a fully humanized IgG1 monoclonal antibody that binds to both soluble and membrane-bound TNF-α. This antibody has greater TNF-α binding affinity than infliximab and adalimumab [115]. This drug was FDA approved for the treatment of ulcerative colitis, RA, PA, and AS in 2013 [116]. The success of other TNF-α inhibitors (adalimumab and infliximab) in the treatment of uveitis paved way for the use of golimumab in uveitis [117]. Retrospective and prospective studies of golimumab in uveitis showed promising results of its effectiveness in maintaining remission. Retrospective analysis of the efficacy of golimumab in patients with recurrent uveitis between 2013 and 2015 showed remission achieved in 12 eyes out of 15 after a median follow-up period of 11 months [118]. A prospective study of 15 patients with refractory uveitis related with spondyloarthritis demonstrated the effectiveness of golimumab in uveitis. The results from this study showed rapid improvement of intraocular inflammation in most of the patients with chronic or relapsing uveitis including patients that were refractory to other TNF-α inhibitors [119].

*Administration and dosing*: Golimumab is marketed under the brand name Simponi (Janssen Biotech, Horsham, PA) and is given subcutaneously at a dose of 50 mg once a month or 200 mg then 100 mg at week 2 and 100 mg every 4 weeks for UC. It can be given intravenously at a dose of 2 mg/kg at week 0 and 4 and then every 8 weeks.

*Adverse effects*: Golimumab as with other TNF-α inhibitors interferes with the inflammatory response, so the use of this drug is associated with side effects similar to those seen in other TNF-α, specifically increased risk of bacterial infections and reactivation of TB [120–122]. When golimumab is combined with antimetabolites such as azathioprine or 6-mercaptopurine, it can lead to an increased risk of malignancies [123]. Please see full prescribing information for complete list.

*Contraindications*: None are listed with the FDA [124]. Tuberculosis reactivation or newly acquired tuberculosis has been reported to have an increased incidence in patients on TNF inhibitors [86, 87]; additional discussion is provided at the end of this section.

## 2.5 Certolizumab

Certolizumab is a member of the TNF-α inhibitors that was developed and approved by the FDA for the treatment of Crohn's disease and RA in 2008 and 2009, respectively [125]. Certolizumab pegol is a humanized antigen-binding fragment (Fab) of monoclonal antibody that targets TNF-α and lacks the Fc region. The Fab fragment is conjugated to polyethylene glycol to increase the half-life of certolizumab compared to other TNF inhibitors [2]. Interest in effectiveness of certolizumab in the treatment of uveitis occurred as an indirect consequence of treatment of systemic diseases associated with uveitis [126]. A retrospective study reported the effectiveness of certolizumab in uveitis, which highlighted the efficacy of certolizumab in five of seven patients with uveitis refractory to other anti-TNF-α agents [126]. Prospective studies are ongoing to test the efficacy of certolizumab in anterior uveitis (NCT03020992 clinicaltrials.gov).

*Administration and dosing*: Certolizumab is marketed under the trade name Cimzia (UCB, Brussels, Belgium). It is administered subcutaneously at a dose of 400 mg at weeks 0, 2, and 4 and then 200–400 mg every 4 weeks.

*Adverse effects*: Studies of the effectiveness of certolizumab in the treatment of autoimmune diseases including uveitis have recorded serious side effects that include new-onset uveitis [127, 128]. Others have observed worsening of arthritis symptoms following treatment with certolizumab. Other serious side effects include increase risk of infection, lupus-like syndrome, and cancer [129]. Please see full prescribing information for complete list.

*Contraindications*: Serious hypersensitivity reaction to certolizumab pegol or the inactive components has been reported [130]. Tuberculosis reactivation or newly acquired tuberculosis has been reported to have an increased incidence in patients on TNF inhibitors [86, 87]; additional discussion is provided at the end of this section.

TNF inhibitors suppress the signals that occur early in the inflammatory cascade and with the exception of etanercept have produced remarkable outcomes in uveitis. Currently, adalimumab and infliximab have been shown to be effective in the treatment of refractory uveitis especially in Behcet's disease-related uveitis or JIA. However, only adalimumab is approved by the FDA for the treatment of uveitis. Because uveitis has occurred in patients being treated with etanercept for autoimmune disease, it is not recommended for the treatment of uveitis [127]. The reactivation of latent tuberculosis or newly acquired tuberculosis is not listed as a contraindication by the FDA, but there are multiple reports that the incidence of tuberculosis reactivation or newly acquired infection is greater in patients on TNF inhibitor therapy [86, 87]. As such, tuberculosis screening before initiation of TNF inhibitor therapy and routine screening for tuberculosis are highly recommended. Additional clinical outcome data from large population studies will be required to demonstrate the safety and efficacy of golimumab and certolizumab. The effectiveness and utilization of TNF-α inhibitors in the treatment of uveitis are limited by the huge cost of these drugs, limited outcome data on clinical use of TNF-α inhibitors in some disease-specific uveitis, and severe side effects in some cases.

## 3. IL-1 inhibitors

The biological agents classified as IL-1 inhibitors target and inhibit the proinflammatory cytokine, IL-1β, and its receptor, IL-1R. IL-1 is a strong proinflammatory cytokine that plays a role in both local and systemic immune responses and is also involved in tissue damage during chronic inflammation [131, 132]. IL-1 mediates its inflammatory response through IL-1α and IL-1β. The latter has been reported to be a critical mediator of autoimmunity when compared with IL-1α [133]. IL-1β is secreted by innate immune cells such as macrophages, neutrophils, dendritic cells, and vascular endothelial cells [55]. IL-1β signals through the IL-1 receptor (IL-1R) to produce its inflammatory effects such as differentiation and expansion of antigen-specific T cells, cell maturation, and induction of acute-phase reaction [134]. This cytokine signaling is known to play a role in autoimmune diseases as demonstrated clinically with significantly elevated levels of IL-1β in biological samples including tears of uveitis patients compared to healthy controls [135]. Also, high levels of this cytokine are implicated in some systemic autoimmune diseases including those associated with uveitis [131].

Studies have shown that loss of IL-1 signaling provides protection from uveitis in animal models of autoimmune uveitis [131]. Being a pleiotropic cytokine, IL-1 activity is tightly regulated by a naturally occurring antagonist of IL-1 receptor (IL-1RA) which specifically inhibits the activities of IL-1 cytokines through blockade of IL-1 receptor. Under physiologic conditions, balance exists between the specific receptor antagonist and IL-1. However, imbalance in the levels of IL-1 and/or IL-1 RA can increase the risk of developing immune-mediated diseases [136]. Also, exogenous administration of IL-1RA in animal models showed inhibition of IL-1 signaling events [136]. Biological agents such as recombinant IL-1R antagonist (anakinra) which mimics the activity of IL-RA have been developed and have shown great success in the reduction of autoimmune diseases [137, 138]. Other biological agents such as soluble decoy IL-1 receptor (rilonacept) and neutralizing monoclonal antibodies (canakinumab and gevokizumab) that have specific inhibition of IL-1 activity have also been utilized in the treatment of autoimmune diseases. Suppression of ocular inflammation may be achieved due to the efficacy of IL-1β inhibitors in the control of inflammation in systemic autoimmune diseases that are associated with uveitis. Additional discussion of these inhibitors is provided below.

## 3.1 Anakinra

Anakinra was first introduced in 1993 (Kineret, Amgen Inc., Thousand Oaks, California), and it is a recombinant non-glycosylated human IL-1RA. It was first approved for the treatment of RA and neonatal-onset multisystem inflammatory disease (NOMID) by the FDA in 2001 [139]. There is limited data on the use of anakinra in the treatment of uveitis; however, a few case studies have reported its effectiveness in uveitis. One study looked at its effect as a treatment for NOMID, which is associated with childhood uveitis; anakinra produced resolution of ocular symptoms in addition to the systemic disease improvement. In this case study, a 4-year-old with chronic infantile neurological cutaneous articular (CINCA) syndrome that is associated with uveitis, who had a poor response to TNF-α inhibitors, showed a significant sustained improvement with anakinra [140]. Another case series also demonstrated the effectiveness of anakinra in two patients with anterior uveitis due to exposure to etanercept or uveitis refractory to infliximab [141]. Also, a retrospective study of 19 patients with Behcet's disease-related uveitis showed effective control of inflammation and improvement in ocular symptoms after 12 months of treatment with anakinra [142].

*Administration and dosing*: Anakinra is sold under the brand name Kineret (Swedish Orphan Biovitrum Stockholm, Sweden) and is given subcutaneously at a dose of 100 mg daily or up to 8 mg/kg a day.

*Adverse effects*: Anakinra is associated with side effect that ranges from a local reaction at the injection site to more severe side effects such as hepatitis, neutropenia, and increase risk of infection [143–145]. Another side effect that could occur is the generation of autoantibodies against anakinra [146]. Please see full prescribing information for complete list.

*Contraindications*: Serious hypersensitivity reaction to *E. coli*-derived proteins, Kineret, or the inactive components [147].

## 3.2 Canakinumab

Canakinumab is a human monoclonal antibody against IL-1β that was first approved by the FDA in 2009 for the treatment of cryopyrin-associated periodic syndromes (CAPS), and, subsequently, it was approved for the treatment of SJIA and JIA in 2013 [148, 149]. Canakinumab inhibits IL-1β by directly binding and neutralizing IL-1β signaling. The long-term effectiveness of canakinumab as a treatment for uveitis has not been studied. However, several case studies show canakinumab as a potential therapeutic for refractory uveitis. Successful resolution of inflammation with canakinumab treatment was seen in a case report of a 64-year-old patient with CAPS-associated uveitis [150]. Another case series by Brambilla et al. (2016) showed successful treatment of refractory uveitis with canakinumab in two children. The first patient in this study was a 9-year-old with recurrent uveitis associated with JIA intolerant to TNF-α inhibitors and refractory to other immune modulatory drugs. Clinical improvement was achieved within 12 months of initiating canakinumab [25]. The second patient, a 6-year-old boy with bilateral uveitis refractory to TNF-α inhibitors, showed a faster responsiveness with remarkable improvement to canakinumab within 2 months of treatment [25]. Another case study of a 16-year-old with severe Behcet's disease associated refractory panuveitis, responded to a single dose of canakinumab with remission of uveitis for at least 8 weeks [151]. Overall, the case series provides evidence of the effectiveness of canakinumab for the treatment of uveitis. In addition, a retrospective study of 19 patients with BD-related uveitis showed an improvement of ocular symptoms after 12 months of treatment with canakinumab [142].

Additional prospective and retrospective studies in large patient groups are needed to validate the effects of canakinumab in uveitis.

*Administration and dosing*: Canakinumab is marketed as Ilaris (Novartis, East Hanover, NJ) and given at a dose of 150–300 mg subcutaneously every 4 weeks or 2–4 mg/kg every 4 weeks.

*Adverse effects*: Side effects of this drug include an increased risk of infection [152, 153]. Please see full prescribing information for complete list.

*Contraindications*: Serious hypersensitivity to Ilaris or the inactive components [154].

### 3.3 Gevokizumab

Gevokizumab is a humanized recombinant IgG2 monoclonal antibody with high affinity for IL-1β. Its ability to bind strongly to IL-1β prompted interest in its use as a biological agent for autoimmune uveitis. A prospective study of eight patients with anterior scleritis showed improvement in symptoms in seven of the patients following treatment with 60 mg SC of gevokizumab every 4 weeks for 12 weeks and continued to show improvement for 36 more weeks [155].

Gul et al. conducted a prospective study to test the efficacy of gevokizumab in patients with acute exacerbation of resistant uveitis in Behcet's disease. Seven adult patients were given a single intravenous gevokizumab infusion at a dose of 0.3 mg/kg. All patients experienced a rapid clinical response and resolution of intraocular inflammation within a median duration of 14 days [156]. Gul et al. also conducted another prospective study to test the efficacy and safety of gevokizumab in 21 patients with Behcet's disease-related uveitis; 3 patients were withdrawn from the study due to exacerbation of uveitis, but 14 patients showed responsiveness within 21 days [157]. These studies provide evidence of the effectiveness of gevokizumab in uveitis, especially the Behcet's-related uveitis. However, the EYEGUARD clinical trials did not show efficacy of gevokizumab in the treatment of uveitis [158]. In the EYEGUARD study, 83 patients with Behcet's disease-related uveitis were recruited into the study. Study groups were given 60 mg of gevokizumab every 4 weeks subcutaneously and were well tolerated. However, the results from this study did not show any treatment efficacy of gevokizumab compared to the placebo group [158]. The conflicting results from these two studies may be due to the route of administration with intravenous infusion being superior to subcutaneous administration. As such, further studies on the dosage, long-term efficacy, and safety of gevokizumab for uveitis treatment are necessary.

*Administration and dosing*: XOMA 052 (XOMA Corporation, Berkeley, CA, USA) is the brand name of gevokizumab. It has not been FDA approved but in trials has been administered at a dose of 60 mg IV or SC every 4 weeks.

*Adverse effects*: Gevokizumab is generally tolerated; however, it can result in mild side effects that include injection site reaction, neutropenia, and hypoglycemia [155, 159]. Please see full prescribing information for complete list.

*Contraindications*: None are listed with the FDA because it is not yet FDA approved.

### 3.4 Rilonacept

Rilonacept is a fully humanized IL-1 fusion protein, and it consists of the ligand-binding domain of the extracellular component of the IL-1 receptor and IL-1 receptor accessory protein. Rilonacept binds to IL-1β to prevent it from interacting with IL-1 receptor, thus preventing IL-1 signaling. This drug is FDA approved for the treatment of autoinflammatory diseases such as familial cold autoinflammatory syndrome (FCAS) and Muckle-Wells syndrome (MWS) [160]. However, there are no clinical data on the use of rilonacept in uveitis, but it is currently being evaluated as a treatment for uveitis [161].

*Administration and dosing*: Rilonacept is marketed as Arcalyst by Regeneron Pharmaceuticals, Tarrytown, New York. It is given subcutaneously at a dose of two 160 mg injections at week 0 and then 160 mg/week.

*Adverse effects*: Local and/or hypersensitivity reaction [162, 163]. Other side effects reported include gastrointestinal bleeding and an increased risk for *Streptococcus pneumoniae* meningitis [160]. Please see full prescribing information for complete list.

Some autoimmune diseases such as rheumatic diseases respond to IL-1β inhibitors. However, the effects of these biologics in uveitis are not conclusive. Some IL-1β inhibitors such as anakinra have demonstrated efficacy in Behcet's disease-related uveitis and autoinflammatory diseases such as NOMID that could be associated with uveitis [139]. Additional large clinical studies are required to evaluate the efficacy of IL-1β as a therapy for autoimmune uveitis.

*Contraindications*: None listed with the FDA [164].

## 4. IL-6 inhibitors

IL-6 is a powerful proinflammatory cytokine that is secreted by both innate and adaptive immune cells (B and T cells). Due to its pleiotropic effects including T-cell activation, IL-6 is implicated in many T-cell-mediated diseases [7]. Biological agents that inhibit IL-6 have been used as a treatment for autoimmune diseases such as RA and JIA. In spite of the proinflammatory effects, it has a role in tumor survival, so blockage of IL-6 is also effective as a cancer treatment, particularly large-cell lung cancer and ovarian cancer [165].

### 4.1 Tocilizumab

Tocilizumab is a fully humanized monoclonal antibody against both soluble and membrane-bound IL-6 receptors. It is currently FDA approved for the treatment of SJIA and RA, and it has profoundly improved disease outcomes [166]. A study by Tappeiner et al. has reported that two out of three patients with JIA-related uveitis responded to tocilizumab that was refractory to anti-TNF-α therapy [167]. Furthermore, a retrospective study that analyzed disease outcomes in five patients with refractory uveitis showed sustained remission after a mean follow-up period of 8.4 months [168]. A similar outcome was observed in another study testing the efficacy of tocilizumab to treat refractory uveitis with 10 out of 17 patients responding to IL-6 blockade [169]. A prospective STOP-UVEITIS study to test the safety, tolerability, and efficacy of tocilizumab in 37 patients with noninfectious uveitis was conducted by Quan et al. (2017); the result of this study shows tolerance at 6 months of drug initiation [170]. These studies and several case studies have reported that tocilizumab may be effective in the treatment of refractory uveitis [171, 172]. Also, Ruiz-Medrano et al. compiled data on the use of tocilizumab in the treatment of ocular conditions between 2011 and 2017. They found that tocilizumab is effective in the treatment of variety of ocular inflammatory conditions including refractory uveitis [173].

*Administration and dosing*: Tocilizumab (Actemra, Genentech, South San Francisco, CA, USA) is typically administered at a dose of 4–12 mg/kg every 2–4 weeks when given intravenously and 162 every 1–2 weeks when given subcutaneously.

*Adverse effects*: Side effects from Actemra include neutropenia with increased risk of fungal and bacterial infections and opportunistic infections [174]. Other side effects include hypersensitivity, increased risk of gastric perforation, and malignancies [175–177]. Please see full prescribing information for complete list.

*Contraindications*: Hypersensitivity to Actemra [178]. Tuberculosis reactivation has been reported in patients undergoing IL-6 inhibitor therapy [179], so patients should be initially tested for latent tuberculosis and should be routinely monitored for newly acquired tuberculosis.

| Biological Target/ Pathway | Generic name | Brand name | Specific Target | Company | Route | Manufacturer Suggested Dose | Indications (FDA approved) | FDA approved for uveitis |
|---|---|---|---|---|---|---|---|---|
| TNF-α | Etanercept | Enbrel | soluble TNF-α and β | Amgen, Thousand Oaks, CA | SC | 50 mg every 1-2 week(s) or 0.8 mg/kg weekly | RA, PA, PP, JIA, AS | Not recommended for Uveitis |
| | Adalimumab | Humira | TNF-α | Abbvie Inc., North Chicago, IL. | SC | 40-80 mg every 1- 2 week(s) | RA, JIA, PA, AS, Crohn's, UC, PP, HS, uveitis | Approved for uveitis, 2016 |
| | Infliximab | Remicade | TNF-α | Janssen Biotech Inc., PA | IV | 3-5 mg/kg every 2 weeks for 6 weeks then once every 8 weeks | Crohn's, UC, RA, AS, PA, PP | Not FDA approved for Uveitis |
| | Golimumab | Simponi | TNF-α | Janssen Biotech Inc., PA | SC or IV | SC: 50 mg once a month; 200 mg then 100 mg at week 2, and 100 mg every four weeks for UC IV: 2 mg/kg at week 0 and 4, then every 8 weeks | UC (not for IV), RA, PA, AS | Not FDA approved for Uveitis |
| | Certolizumab pegol | Cimzia | TNF-α | UCB Pharma Inc., Brussels, Belgium | SC | 400 mg every 2 weeks for 4 weeks then 200-400 mg every 2-4 weeks | Crohn's disease, RA, PA, AS, PP | Not FDA approved for Uveitis |
| IL-1β | Anakinra | Kineret | IL-1β | Swedish Orphan Biovitrum, Sweden | SC | 100 mg daily or up to 8 mg/kg daily | RA, NOMID, CAPS | Not FDA approved for uveitis |
| | Canakinumab | ILaris | IL-1β | Novartis, Basel, Switzerland | SC | 150-300 mg once a month or 2-4 mg/kg every 4 weeks | CAPS, TRAPS, HIDS/MKD, FMF | Not FDA approved for Uveitis |
| | Gevokizumab | XOMA 052 | IL-1β | Novartis, Basel, Switzerland | SC or IV | 60 mg /month | In development | Not FDA approved for Uveitis |
| | Rilonacept | Arcalyst | IL-1β | Regeneron, Tarrytown, New York | SC | 160 mg/week with 320 mg loading dose at week 0 | CAPS, FCAS, MWS | Not FDA approved for uveitis |
| IL-6 | Tocilizumab | Actemra | IL-6 receptor | Genetech Inc., CA | IV or SC | IV: 4-12 mg/kg every 2-4 weeks SC: 162 mg every 1-2 week(s) | GCA, SJIA, RA, PJIA, cytokine release syndrome | Not FDA approved for uveitis |
| | Sarilumab | Kevzara | IL-6 receptor | Regeneron/Sanofi NY | SC | 200 mg every 2 weeks | RA | Not FDA approved for uveitis |
| | Olokizumab | Not yet assigned | IL-6 | UCB Pharma Inc., Belgium / Licensed to R-Pharma, Moscow, Russia | SC | 64 mg every 2 or 4 weeks | RA - Clinical trial NCT0276036 8 to be completed January 2019 | Not FDA approved for uveitis |
| | Clazakizumab | Not yet assigned | IL-6 | Vitaeris, Vancouver, Canada | SC | 5- 25 mg | In development | Not FDA approved for uveitis |
| | Siltuximab | Sylvant | IL-6 | Janssen Biotech, PA | IV | 11 mg/kg every 3 weeks | Castleman's disease | Not FDA approved for uveitis |
| IL-17 | Secukinumab | Cosentyx | IL-17A | Novartis, Basel, Switzerland | SC | 150-300 mg weekly for 4 weeks, then once a month | PP, AS, PA | Not FDA approved for uveitis |
| | Ixekizumab | Taltz | IL-17A | Eli Lilly and Co, Indianapolis, IN | SC | 160 mg every 2 weeks for 3 months then 80 mg once a month or 160 mg at week 0 then 80 mg every 4 weeks | PP, PA | Not FDA approved for uveitis |
| | Brodalumab | Siliq | IL-17 receptor | Bausch Health, Laval, Canada | SC | 210 mg weekly for 3 weeks then once every 2 weeks | PP | Not FDA approved for uveitis |

**Table 1.**
*List of biologics discussed in sections 3–6.*

### 4.2 Sarilumab

Sarilumab is another IL-6 receptor inhibitor, it is a fully humanized monoclonal antibody against the alpha subunit of the IL-6 receptor, and in 2017 it was FDA approved as a treatment for RA [180]. Sarilumab has shown some potential as an effective therapy for autoimmune uveitis in a prospective SATURN study [181]. In this randomized study, 57 patients with posterior uveitis on steroids with or without methotrexate were treated with 200 mg of sarilumab or placebo every 2 weeks. About 64% of the patients on sarilumab showed clinical improvement and steroid-sparing effects at 16 weeks after treatment initiation [181].

*Administration and dosing*: Sarilumab is marketed as Kevzara (Regeneron/Sanofi Tarrytown, NY, USA), and in the treatment of RA, sarilumab is typically given at 200 mg SC every 2 weeks.

*Adverse effects*: Increased risk of GI perforation and hepatitis [182]. Please see full prescribing information for complete list.

*Contraindications*: Hypersensitivity to Kevzara or the inactive ingredients [183]. Tuberculosis reactivation has been reported in patients undergoing IL-6 inhibitor therapy [179], so patients should be initially tested for latent tuberculosis and should be routinely monitored for newly acquired tuberculosis.

*Other IL-6 inhibitors*: Olokizumab (UCB, Brussels, Belgium) and clazakizumab (Alder Biopharma, Bothell, WA, USA) are currently being evaluated in clinical trials for the treatment of autoimmune diseases (which can be associated with uveitis) such as RA. Siltuximab (Janssen, Horsham, PA, USA) has been FDA approved for the treatment of Castleman's disease [184–187]. However, there are little or no data regarding the efficacy of these drugs in uveitis. See **Table 1** for additional information regarding these drugs.

## 5. IL-17 inhibitors

IL-17 is a proinflammatory cytokine produced by Th17 cells, a subset of inflammatory T cells, involved in an inflammatory response to self and certain extracellular bacteria and fungi. While IL-17 can be produced by other cells, it is the characteristic cytokine produced by Th17 cells. IL-17 is involved in the recruitment and activation of neutrophils [188, 189]. Animal and human studies have elucidated the critical role of IL-17 in the pathogenesis of autoimmune diseases including uveitis [190, 191]. Inhibitors of IL-17 have produced remarkable improvement in the outcome of autoimmune diseases especially rheumatoid diseases [192]. IL-17 inhibitors such as secukinumab (AIN457), ixekizumab (Taltz), and brodalumab (AMG 827) are FDA approved for the treatment of severe psoriasis [193]. Knowledge of the efficacies of these biological agents in autoimmune diseases provides the potential for use in uveitis, especially uveitis that is refractory to conventional drugs and other biologics. Blockade of IL-17 in animal models of autoimmune uveitis has produced significant improvement in uveitis symptoms [194].

### 5.1 Secukinumab

Secukinumab is a fully humanized monoclonal antibody that neutralizes IL-17A. It is FDA approved for treatment of moderate to severe plaque psoriasis [195]. Hueber et al. tested the efficacy of AIN457 in a prospective study with 104 uveitis patients, RA or psoriasis. About 50% of the uveitis patients showed a rapid response within 2 weeks and by 8 weeks of drug initiation; 13 out of 16 patients responded to AIN457 [196]. In a prospective study of 118 patients with Behcet's disease (SHIELD study), the rate of recurrent ocular exacerbation of uveitis did not differ between the patients that received secukinumab or placebo. The study concluded that secukinumab did not demonstrate efficacy in the treatment of uveitis. Similar outcomes were concluded from the INSURE and ENDURE studies in which altering the dosing schedule of secukinumab did not improve the efficacy of secukinumab in uveitis patients [197, 198]. The outcome of these studies may have differed from the initial report by Hueber et al. because the differences were noted in the patient disease profile, concomitant immunosuppressive therapies, and route of administration [197]. One prospective study demonstrated that intravenous secukinumab (10 mg/kg or 30 mg/kg) had better efficacy than subcutaneous secukinumab (300 mg). Therefore, these studies demonstrate that patients responded better to secukinumab when it was administered IV [198].

*Administration and dosing*: Secukinumab was initially named AIN 457 and has been renamed Cosentyx (Novartis). It is given subcutaneously for plaque psoriasis at a dose of 150–300 mg weekly for 4 weeks and then every 4 weeks. However, it has been suggested that it is more effective given IV at 30 mg/kg for the treatment of noninfectious uveitis [198].

*Adverse effects*: Cosentyx is associated with an increased risk of infection, hypersensitivity reaction, and inflammatory bowel disease [199, 200]. Please see full prescribing information for complete list.

*Contraindications*: Hypersensitivity to Cosentyx or any of the inactive ingredients [201]. Tuberculosis reactivation is listed as a warning by the FDA, but it has been reported in a multicenter retrospective study by Novartis [202] and in a review of the literature [203] that there is no increased risk of tuberculosis reactivation.

Other IL-17 inhibitors: Additional biologics that target the IL-17 pathway include ixekizumab and brodalumab. Ixekizumab targets IL-17A and is FDA approved to treat plaque psoriasis and psoriatic arthritis. Brodalumab targets the IL-17 receptor and is FDA approved for the treatment of plaque psoriasis. At the time of this review, clinical trials for uveitis are underway, so there are no clinical reports regarding their efficacy in autoimmune uveitis. See **Table 1** for additional information regarding these drugs.

## 6. Other biologics

Biological agents that target and inhibit cytokines such as TNF-α and IL-1β have been extensively studied and have resulted in improving clinical outcomes in many autoimmune diseases including uveitis. We chose to include a more in-depth discussion of biologics that target IL-6 and IL-17 because IL-6 is such a central inflammatory cytokine that bridges both innate and adaptive immunities, and IL-17 is the characteristic cytokine produced by Th17 T cells that are involved in autoimmune diseases. The efficacies of these biological agents have spurred the introduction of additional biologics that target other inflammatory mediators implicated in autoimmunity. Also, the heterogeneity of uveitis, non-responsiveness or adverse effects associated with the current biologics used for the treatment of uveitis, provides the need to examine the efficacy of other biological agents that target other mediators implicated in autoimmunity. Recombinant interferon and IVIG are biologics used for the treatment of refractory autoimmune uveitis and other inflammatory conditions [204–206]. However, the precise mechanism of action for these medications is not well understood. Rituximab targets CD20 on B cells and is used for the treatment of ocular cicatricial pemphigoid, scleritis, and uveitis associated with granulomatosis with polyangiitis [207, 208]. There are also additional biologics that target specific cytokines and cell surface proteins that are in development and undergoing clinical trials for autoimmune diseases that may include uveitis, rheumatoid arthritis, ulcerative colitis, psoriatic arthritis, and others. Since these other biologics are still in various phases of development, we will not go into the same level of detail as in the others discussed above. Because there are many medications that are not public knowledge, the following is not an exhaustive list. Some of the medications that may be available for the treatment of autoimmune uveitis in the near future target IL-15, IL-23 p40, interferon, and its receptors, CD52, CD4, VEGF, and VCAM. A fusion protein consisting of the B7-binding portion of CTLA4 and IgG is also available and is being evaluated for the treatment of autoimmune uveitis.

## 7. Switching biological therapies

The development of multiple biologics that target specific inflammatory pathways has greatly increased the treatment options available for patients with autoimmune uveitis. With so many options available, it is of interest to determine if there is an advantage to switching the biologic, either within the same class or to a different class. Large clinical studies have not been done with uveitis cohorts, but some have been done with rheumatoid arthritis patients. There is some evidence that switching biologics within the same class, specifically related to TNF-α inhibitors, for reasons related to adverse reactions rather than efficacy may be beneficial [209]. A more recent study found that switching from TNF-α inhibitors to another biological class showed a significantly greater benefit than switching to another TNF-α inhibitor [210]. Therefore, it is still not clear which is the best biological treatment strategy for autoimmune uveitis patients, but there is some indication based on RA patients that switching to a different class of biologics may have significantly better outcomes than switching to another biological within the same class.

## 8. Conclusions

In this review, we focus on biologics that target TNF-α, IL-β, IL-6, and IL-17. The rationale for this is that TNF-α, IL-β, and IL-6 cytokines are involved in key inflammatory pathways that target both the innate and adaptive arms of the immune response. We also include a brief discussion of IL-17 because it is produced by a specific T-cell subset, and Th17 cells have been demonstrated to be involved in autoimmune diseases [190, 191]. There are other biologics that target other cytokines and cell types, but these are in earlier phases of development and are not yet FDA approved. Additional options for therapy are constantly being studied. Biologics are a newer class of therapeutics that have the advantage over other medications in that they are extremely specific for one target molecule. This specificity makes them attractive as therapeutics because specific pathways and/or cell types can be blocked. Inhibition of a specific pathway or cell type has the advantage over other immunosuppressive therapies that suppress all leukocytes and lymphocytes. A drawback to biologics is the high economic burden associated with these drugs. Because of the high cost associated with biologics, it can be difficult to obtain insurance coverage until multiple therapies have failed. As such, the cost to the patient could be a permanent loss of vision with repeated relapses and the use of corticosteroids while transitioning to a new therapy. Importantly, because these therapies have efficacy in treatment of systemic autoimmune diseases such as RA, inflammatory bowel diseases, and Behcet's disease with a uveitis manifestation they may be effective for the majority of uveitis patients that only have ocular involvement [2, 211]. Therefore, additional appropriately powered clinical studies are necessary to demonstrate the effectiveness of biologics for the treatment of chronic autoimmune uveitis.

## Acknowledgements

Funding was provided by the National Institutes of Health/National Eye Institute grant EY024951 and in part by an unrestricted Research to Prevent Blindness grant (New York, NY, USA).

## Conflict of interest declaration

The authors have no conflicts of interest to disclose.

## List of abbreviations

| | |
|---|---|
| APCs | antigen-presenting cells |
| AS | ankylosing spondylitis |
| AU | autoimmune uveitis |
| BD | Behcet's disease |
| CAPS | cryopyrin-associated periodic syndromes |
| CINCA | chronic infantile neurological cutaneous articular |
| CLL | chronic lymphocytic leukemia |
| FCAS | familial cold autoinflammatory syndrome |
| FDA | Food and Drug Administration |
| FMF | familial Mediterranean fever |
| GCA | giant cell arteritis |
| HIDS | hyperimmunoglobulin D syndrome |
| HLA | human leukocyte antigen |
| HS | hidradenitis suppurativa |
| IgG | immunoglobulin G |
| IL-17 | interleukin-17 |
| IL-1b | interleukin-1 beta |
| IL-6 | interleukin-6 |
| JIA | juvenile idiopathic arthritis |
| MKD | mevalonate kinase deficiency |
| MS | multiple sclerosis |
| mTOR | mammalian target of rapamycin |
| MWS | Muckle-Wells syndrome |
| NHL | non-Hodgkin lymphoma |
| NOMID | neonatal-onset multisystem inflammatory disease |
| NSAIDs | nonsteroidal anti-inflammatory drugs |
| PA | psoriatic arthritis |
| PJIA | polyarticular juvenile idiopathic arthritis |
| PP | plaque psoriasis |
| RA | rheumatoid arthritis |
| SJIA | systemic juvenile idiopathic arthritis |

| | |
|---|---|
| TLR | toll-like receptor |
| TNF-a | tumor necrosis factor-alpha |
| TRAPS | tumor necrosis factor receptor-associated periodic syndrome |
| UC | ulcerative colitis |

## Author details

Ashvini Reddy[1], Fauziyya Muhammad[2] and Darren J. Lee[3]*

1 Department of Ophthalmology, Dean McGee Eye Institute, University of Oklahoma Health Sciences Center, Oklahoma City, Oklahoma, USA

2 Department of Microbiology and Immunology, University of Oklahoma Health Sciences Center, Oklahoma City, Oklahoma, USA

3 Department of Ophthalmology, Dean McGee Eye Institute, Department of Microbiology and Immunology, University of Oklahoma Health Sciences Center, Oklahoma City, Oklahoma, USA

*Address all correspondence to: darren-lee@ouhsc.edu

## References

[1] Lee DJ, Taylor AW. Following EAU recovery there is an associated MC5r-dependent APC induction of regulatory immunity in the spleen. Investigative Ophthalmology & Visual Science. 2011; **52**:8862-8867

[2] Pasadhika S, Rosenbaum JT. Update on the use of systemic biologic agents in the treatment of noninfectious uveitis. Biologics. 2014;**8**:67-81

[3] Jabs DA, Nussenblatt RB, Rosenbaum JT, Standardization of Uveitis Nomenclature Working G. Standardization of uveitis nomenclature for reporting clinical data. Results of the First International Workshop. American Journal of Ophthalmology. 2005;**140**: 509-516

[4] Lerman MA, Rabinovich CE. The future is now: Biologics for non-infectious pediatric anterior uveitis. Paediatric Drugs. 2015;**17**:283-301

[5] Brezin AP. Semiology and classification of uveitis. La Revue du Praticien. 1999;**49**:1982-1988

[6] Rathinam SR, Babu M. Algorithmic approach in the diagnosis of uveitis. Indian Journal of Ophthalmology. 2013; **61**:255-262

[7] Barry RJ, Nguyen QD, Lee RW, Murray PI, Denniston AK. Pharmacotherapy for uveitis: Current management and emerging therapy. Clinical Ophthalmology. 2014;**8**: 1891-1911

[8] Curnow SJ, Scheel-Toellner D, Jenkinson W, Raza K, Durrani OM, Faint JM, et al. Inhibition of T cell apoptosis in the aqueous humor of patients with uveitis by IL-6/soluble IL-6 receptor trans-signaling. Journal of Immunology. 2004;**173**:5290-5297

[9] Durrani OM, Tehrani NN, Marr JE, Moradi P, Stavrou P, Murray PI. Degree, duration, and causes of visual loss in uveitis. The British Journal of Ophthalmology. 2004;**88**:1159-1162

[10] Suttorp-Schulten MS, Rothova A. The possible impact of uveitis in blindness: A literature survey. The British Journal of Ophthalmology. 1996; **80**:844-848

[11] You C, Sahawneh HF, Ma L, Kubaisi B, Schmidt A, Foster CS. A review and update on orphan drugs for the treatment of noninfectious uveitis. Clinical Ophthalmology. 2017;**11**:257-265

[12] Babu K, Mahendradas P. Medical management of uveitis - current trends. Indian Journal of Ophthalmology. 2013; **61**:277-283

[13] Suhler EB, Thorne JE, Mittal M, Betts KA, Tari S, Camez A, et al. Corticosteroid-related adverse events systematically increase with corticosteroid dose in noninfectious intermediate, posterior, or panuveitis: Post hoc analyses from the VISUAL-1 and VISUAL-2 trials. Ophthalmology. 2017;**12**:1799-1807

[14] Merida S, Palacios E, Navea A, Bosch-Morell F. New immunosuppressive therapies in uveitis treatment. International Journal of Molecular Sciences. 2015;**16**:18778-18795

[15] Smith JR. Management of uveitis. Clinical and Experimental Medicine. 2004;**4**:21-29

[16] Hunter RS, Lobo AM. Dexamethasone intravitreal implant for the treatment of noninfectious uveitis. Clinical Ophthalmology. 2011;**5**: 1613-1621

[17] Jabs DA, Rosenbaum JT, Foster CS, Holland GN, Jaffe GJ, Louie JS, et al. Guidelines for the use of immunosuppressive drugs in patients with ocular inflammatory disorders: Recommendations of an expert panel. American Journal of Ophthalmology. 2000;**130**:492-513

[18] Jabs DA. Immunosuppression for the uveitides. Ophthalmology. 2018;**125**: 193-202

[19] Allison AC, Eugui EM. Mycophenolate mofetil and its mechanisms of action. Immunopharmacology. 2000;**47**:85-118

[20] Arellano B, Graber DJ, Sentman CL. Regulatory T cell-based therapies for autoimmunity. Discovery Medicine. 2016;**22**:73-80

[21] Dejaco C, Duftner C, Grubeck-Loebenstein B, Schirmer M. Imbalance of regulatory T cells in human autoimmune diseases. Immunology. 2006;**117**:289-300

[22] Li J, Kim SG, Blenis J. Rapamycin: One drug, many effects. Cell Metabolism. 2014;**19**:373-379

[23] Imrie FR, Dick AD. Biologics in the treatment of uveitis. Current Opinion in Ophthalmology. 2007;**18**:481-486

[24] Levy-Clarke G, Jabs DA, Read RW, Rosenbaum JT, Vitale A, Van Gelder RN. Expert panel recommendations for the use of anti-tumor necrosis factor biologic agents in patients with ocular inflammatory disorders. Ophthalmology. 2014;**121**:785-796.e3

[25] Brambilla A, Caputo R, Cimaz R, Simonini G. Canakinumab for childhood sight-threatening refractory uveitis: A case series. The Journal of Rheumatology. 2016;**43**:1445-1447

[26] Jaffe GJ, Dick AD, Brezin AP, Nguyen QD, Thorne JE, Kestelyn P, et al. Adalimumab in patients with active noninfectious uveitis. The New England Journal of Medicine. 2016;**375**: 932-943

[27] Barisani-Asenbauer T, Maca SM, Mejdoubi L, Emminger W, Machold K, Auer H. Uveitis–A rare disease often associated with systemic diseases and infections- a systematic review of 2619 patients. Orphanet Journal of Rare Diseases. 2012;7:57

[28] Wildner G, Diedrichs-Mohring M. Autoimmune uveitis induced by molecular mimicry of peptides from rotavirus, bovine casein and retinal S-antigen. European Journal of Immunology. 2003;**33**:2577-2587

[29] Cusick MF, Libbey JE, Fujinami RS. Molecular mimicry as a mechanism of autoimmune disease. Clinical Reviews in Allergy and Immunology. 2012;**42**: 102-111

[30] Willermain F, Rosenbaum JT, Bodaghi B, Rosenzweig HL, Childers S, Behrend T, et al. Interplay between innate and adaptive immunity in the development of non-infectious uveitis. Progress in Retinal and Eye Research. 2012;**31**:182-194

[31] Caspi RR. Understanding autoimmune uveitis through animal models. The Friedenwald Lecture. Investigative Ophthalmology & Visual Science. 2011;**52**:1872-1879

[32] Feltkamp TE. HLA and uveitis. International Ophthalmology. 1990;**14**: 327-333

[33] Shenavandeh S, Jahanshahi KA, Aflaki E, Tavassoli A. Frequency of HLA-B5, HLA-B51 and HLA-B27 in patients with idiopathic uveitis and Behcet's disease: A case-control study. Reumatologia. 2018;**56**:67-72

[34] Caspi RR. A look at autoimmunity and inflammation in the eye. The

Journal of Clinical Investigation. 2010; **120**:3073-3083

[35] Martin TM, Rosenbaum JT. An update on the genetics of HLA B27-associated acute anterior uveitis. Ocular Immunology and Inflammation. 2011; **19**:108-114

[36] Colmegna I, Cuchacovich R, Espinoza LR. HLA-B27-associated reactive arthritis: Pathogenetic and clinical considerations. Clinical Microbiology Reviews. 2004;**17**:348-369

[37] Takeuchi M, Kastner DL, Remmers EF. The immunogenetics of Behcet's disease: A comprehensive review. Journal of Autoimmunity. 2015;**64**: 137-148

[38] Forrester JV, Kuffova L, Dick AD. Autoimmunity, autoinflammation, and infection in uveitis. American Journal of Ophthalmology. 2018;**189**:77-85

[39] Mattapallil MJ, Sahin A, Silver PB, Sun SH, Chan CC, Remmers EF, et al. Common genetic determinants of uveitis shared with other autoimmune disorders. Journal of Immunology. 2008;**180**:6751-6759

[40] Martin TM, Kurz DE, Rosenbaum JT. Genetics of uveitis. Ophthalmology Clinics of North America. 2003;**16**: 555-565

[41] Bi HS, Liu ZF, Cui Y. Pathogenesis of innate immunity and adaptive immunity in the mouse model of experimental autoimmune uveitis. Journal of the Chinese Medical Association. 2015;**78**:276-282

[42] Huhtinen M, Repo H, Laasila K, Jansson SE, Kautiainen H, Karma A, et al. Systemic inflammation and innate immune response in patients with previous anterior uveitis. The British Journal of Ophthalmology. 2002;**86**: 412-417

[43] Perez VL, Caspi RR. Immune mechanisms in inflammatory and degenerative eye disease. Trends in Immunology. 2015;**36**:354-363

[44] Kasper M, Walscheid K, Laffer B, Bauer D, Busch M, Wildschutz L, et al. The phenotype of monocytes in anterior uveitis depends on the HLA-B27 status. Frontiers in Immunology. 2018;**9**:1773

[45] Horai R, Caspi RR. Cytokines in autoimmune uveitis. Journal of Interferon & Cytokine Research. 2011; **31**:733-744

[46] Caspi RR, Silver PB, Luger D, Tang J, Cortes LM, Pennesi G, et al. Mouse models of experimental autoimmune uveitis. Ophthalmic Research. 2008;**40**: 169-174

[47] Dick AD, Forrester JV, Liversidge J, Cope AP. The role of tumour necrosis factor (TNF-alpha) in experimental autoimmune uveoretinitis (EAU). Progress in Retinal and Eye Research. 2004;**23**:617-637

[48] Weinstein JE, Pepple KL. Cytokines in uveitis. Current Opinion in Ophthalmology. 2018;**29**:267-274

[49] Zhao R, Zhou H, Zhang J, Liu X, Su SB. Interleukin-1beta promotes the induction of retinal autoimmune disease. International Immunopharmacology. 2014;**22**:285-292

[50] Jain A, Pasare C. Innate control of adaptive immunity: Beyond the three-signal paradigm. Journal of Immunology. 2017;**198**:3791-3800

[51] Banyer JL, Hamilton NH, Ramshaw IA, Ramsay AJ. Cytokines in innate and adaptive immunity. Reviews in Immunogenetics. 2000;**2**:359-373

[52] Kuwabara T, Ishikawa F, Kondo M, Kakiuchi T. The role of IL-17 and related cytokines in inflammatory autoimmune

diseases. Mediators of Inflammation. 2017;**2017**:3908061

[53] Jawad S, Liu B, Agron E, Nussenblatt RB, Sen HN. Elevated serum levels of interleukin-17A in uveitis patients. Ocular Immunology and Inflammation. 2013;**21**:434-439

[54] Kuiper JJ, Mutis T, de Jager W, de Groot-Mijnes JD, Rothova A. Intraocular interleukin-17 and proinflammatory cytokines in HLA-A29-associated birdshot chorioretinopathy. American Journal of Ophthalmology. 2011;**152**: 177-182.e1

[55] Ooi KG, Galatowicz G, Calder VL, Lightman SL. Cytokines and chemokines in uveitis: Is there a correlation with clinical phenotype? Clinical Medicine & Research. 2006;**4**: 294-309

[56] He Y, Jia SB, Zhang W, Shi JM. New options for uveitis treatment. International Journal of Ophthalmology. 2013;**6**:702-707

[57] Khalili H, Lee RW, Khaw PT, Brocchini S, Dick AD, Copland DA. An anti-TNF-alpha antibody mimetic to treat ocular inflammation. Scientific Reports. 2016;**6**:36905

[58] Cordero-Coma M, Calleja S, Llorente M, Rodriguez E, Franco M, Ruiz de Morales JG. Serum cytokine profile in adalimumab-treated refractory uveitis patients: Decreased IL-22 correlates with clinical responses. Ocular Immunology and Inflammation. 2013;**21**:212-219

[59] Monaco C, Nanchahal J, Taylor P, Feldmann M. Anti-TNF therapy: Past, present and future. International Immunology. 2015;**27**:55-62

[60] Bradley JR. TNF-mediated inflammatory disease. The Journal of Pathology. 2008;**214**:149-160

[61] Parameswaran N, Patial S. Tumor necrosis factor-alpha signaling in macrophages. Critical Reviews in Eukaryotic Gene Expression. 2010;**20**: 87-103

[62] Butler DM, Maini RN, Feldmann M, Brennan FM. Modulation of proinflammatory cytokine release in rheumatoid synovial membrane cell cultures. Comparison of monoclonal anti TNF-alpha antibody with the interleukin-1 receptor antagonist. European Cytokine Network. 1995;**6**: 225-230

[63] Sugita S, Takase H, Taguchi C, Mochizuki M. The role of soluble TNF receptors for TNF-alpha in uveitis. Investigative Ophthalmology & Visual Science. 2007;**48**:3246-3252

[64] Kollias G, Kontoyiannis D, Douni E, Kassiotis G. The role of TNF/TNFR in organ-specific and systemic autoimmunity: Implications for the design of optimized 'anti-TNF' therapies. Current Directions in Autoimmunity. 2002;**5**:30-50

[65] Agrawal R, Iyer J, Connolly J, Iwata D, Teoh S. Cytokines and biologics in non-infectious autoimmune uveitis: Bench to bedside. Indian Journal of Ophthalmology. 2014;**62**:74-81

[66] Busch M, Bauer D, Hennig M, Wasmuth S, Thanos S, Heiligenhaus A. Effects of systemic and intravitreal TNF-alpha inhibition in experimental autoimmune uveoretinitis. Investigative Ophthalmology & Visual Science. 2013; **54**:39-46

[67] Lis K, Kuzawinska O, Balkowiec-Iskra E. Tumor necrosis factor inhibitors - state of knowledge. Archives of Medical Science. 2014;**10**:1175-1185

[68] Haraoui B, Bykerk V. Etanercept in the treatment of rheumatoid arthritis. Therapeutics and Clinical Risk Management. 2007;**3**:99-105

[69] Ardestani S, Li B, Deskins DL, Wu H, Massion PP, Young PP. Membrane versus soluble isoforms of TNF-alpha exert opposing effects on tumor growth and survival of tumor-associated myeloid cells. Cancer Research. 2013;**73**: 3938-3950

[70] Scott LJ. Etanercept: A review of its use in autoimmune inflammatory diseases. Drugs. 2014;**74**:1379-1410

[71] Reiff A, Takei S, Sadeghi S, Stout A, Shaham B, Bernstein B, et al. Etanercept therapy in children with treatment-resistant uveitis. Arthritis and Rheumatism. 2001;**44**:1411-1415

[72] Quartier P, Taupin P, Bourdeaut F, Lemelle I, Pillet P, Bost M, et al. Efficacy of etanercept for the treatment of juvenile idiopathic arthritis according to the onset type. Arthritis and Rheumatism. 2003;**48**:1093-1101

[73] Smith JA, Thompson DJ, Whitcup SM, Suhler E, Clarke G, Smith S, et al. A randomized, placebo-controlled, double-masked clinical trial of etanercept for the treatment of uveitis associated with juvenile idiopathic arthritis. Arthritis and Rheumatism. 2005;**53**:18-23

[74] Baughman RP, Lower EE, Bradley DA, Raymond LA, Kaufman A. Etanercept for refractory ocular sarcoidosis: Results of a double-blind randomized trial. Chest. 2005;**128**: 1062-1047

[75] Foster CS, Tufail F, Waheed NK, Chu D, Miserocchi E, Baltatzis S, et al. Efficacy of etanercept in preventing relapse of uveitis controlled by methotrexate. Archives of Ophthalmology. 2003;**121**:437-440

[76] Raffeiner B, Ometto F, Bernardi L, Botsios C, Punzi L. Inefficacy or paradoxical effect? Uveitis in ankylosing spondylitis treated with etanercept. Case Reports in Medicine. 2014;**2014**:4

[77] Wendling D, Joshi A, Reilly P, Jalundhwala YJ, Mittal M, Bao Y. Comparing the risk of developing uveitis in patients initiating anti-tumor necrosis factor therapy for ankylosing spondylitis: An analysis of a large US claims database. Current Medical Research and Opinion. 2014;**30**: 2515-2521

[78] Reddy AR, Backhouse OC. Does etanercept induce uveitis? The British Journal of Ophthalmology. 2003;**87**:925

[79] Galor A, Perez VL, Hammel JP, Lowder CY. Differential effectiveness of etanercept and infliximab in the treatment of ocular inflammation. Ophthalmology. 2006;**113**:2317-2323

[80] Lim LL, Fraunfelder FW, Rosenbaum JT. Do tumor necrosis factor inhibitors cause uveitis? A registry-based study. Arthritis and Rheumatism. 2007;**56**:3248-3252

[81] Scheinfeld N. The medical uses and side effects of etanercept with a focus on cutaneous disease. Journal of Drugs in Dermatology. 2004;**3**:653-659

[82] Fallahi-Sichani M, Flynn JL, Linderman JJ, Kirschner DE. Differential risk of tuberculosis reactivation among anti-TNF therapies is due to drug binding kinetics and permeability. Journal of Immunology. 2012;**188**:3169-3178

[83] Ramos-Casals M, Roberto Perez A, Diaz-Lagares C, Cuadrado MJ, Khamashta MA. Autoimmune diseases induced by biological agents: A double-edged sword? Autoimmunity Reviews. 2010;**9**:188-193

[84] Ibrahim WH, Hammoudah M, Akhtar N, Al-Hail H, Deleu D. Central nervous system demyelination associated with etanercept in a 51 years old woman. Libyan Journal of Medicine. 2007;**2**:99-102

[85] ENBREL. FDA Approved Drug Products [Internet]. 2018. Available from: https://www.accessdata.fda.gov/drugsatfda_docs/label/2018/103795s5569lbl.pdf

[86] Salmon-Ceron D, Tubach F, Lortholary O, Chosidow O, Bretagne S, Nicolas N, et al. Drug-specific risk of non-tuberculosis opportunistic infections in patients receiving anti-TNF therapy reported to the 3-year prospective French RATIO registry. Annals of the Rheumatic Diseases. 2011; **70**:616-623

[87] Wallis RS, Broder MS, Wong JY, Hanson ME, Beenhouwer DO. Granulomatous infectious diseases associated with tumor necrosis factor antagonists. Clinical Infectious Diseases. 2004;**38**:1261-1265

[88] Gottlieb AB. Tumor necrosis factor blockade: Mechanism of action. The Journal of Investigative Dermatology. Symposium Proceedings. 2007;**12**:1-4

[89] Reimold AM. The role of adalimumab in rheumatic and autoimmune disorders: Comparison with other biologic agents. Open Access Rheumatology. 2012;**4**:33-47

[90] Sheppard J, Joshi A, Betts KA, Hudgens S, Tari S, Chen N, et al. Effect of adalimumab on visual functioning in patients with noninfectious intermediate uveitis, posterior uveitis, and panuveitis in the VISUAL-1 and VISUAL-2 trials. JAMA Ophthalmology. 2017;**135**:511-518

[91] Perra D, Alba MA, Callejas JL, Mesquida M, Rios-Fernandez R, Adan A, et al. Adalimumab for the treatment of Behcet's disease: Experience in 19 patients. Rheumatology (Oxford). 2012; **51**:1825-1831

[92] van Denderen JC, Visman IM, Nurmohamed MT, Suttorp-Schulten MS, van der Horst-Bruinsma IE. Adalimumab significantly reduces the recurrence rate of anterior uveitis in patients with ankylosing spondylitis. The Journal of Rheumatology. 2014;**41**: 1843-1848

[93] Suhler EB, Lowder CY, Goldstein DA, Giles T, Lauer AK, Kurz PA, et al. Adalimumab therapy for refractory uveitis: Results of a multicentre, open-label, prospective trial. The British Journal of Ophthalmology. 2013;**97**: 481-486

[94] Fabiani C, Vitale A, Emmi G, Vannozzi L, Lopalco G, Guerriero S, et al. Efficacy and safety of adalimumab in Behcet's disease-related uveitis: A multicenter retrospective observational study. Clinical Rheumatology. 2017;**36**: 183-189

[95] Biester S, Deuter C, Michels H, Haefner R, Kuemmerle-Deschner J, Doycheva D, et al. Adalimumab in the therapy of uveitis in childhood. The British Journal of Ophthalmology. 2007; **91**:319-324

[96] Ramanan AV, Dick AD, Jones AP, McKay A, Williamson PR, Compeyrot-Lacassagne S, et al. Adalimumab plus Methotrexate for Uveitis in Juvenile Idiopathic Arthritis. The New England Journal of Medicine. 2017;**376**:1637-1646

[97] LaMattina KC, Goldstein DA. Adalimumab for the treatment of uveitis. Expert Review of Clinical Immunology. 2017;**13**:181-188

[98] Neri P, Lettieri M, Fortuna C, Zucchi M, Manoni M, Celani S, et al. Adalimumab (humira) in ophthalmology: A review of the literature. Middle East African Journal of Ophthalmology. 2010;**17**:290-296

[99] Alnasser Alsukhni R, Jriekh Z, Aboras Y. Adalimumab induced or provoked MS in patient with autoimmune uveitis: A case report and

review of the literature. Case Reports in Medicine. 2016;**2016**:1423131

[100] Sim JK, Lee SY, Shim JJ, Kang KH. Pulmonary sarcoidosis induced by adalimumab: A case report and literature review. Yonsei Medical Journal. 2016;**57**:272-273

[101] Humira. FDA Approved Drug Products [Internet]. 2018. Available from: https://www.accessdata.fda.gov/drugsatfda_docs/label/2018/125057s409lbl.pdf

[102] Kaymakcalan Z, Sakorafas P, Bose S, Scesney S, Xiong L, Hanzatian DK, et al. Comparisons of affinities, avidities, and complement activation of adalimumab, infliximab, and etanercept in binding to soluble and membrane tumor necrosis factor. Clinical Immunology. 2009;**131**:308-316

[103] Bickston SJ. Infliximab for ulcerative colitis induction of remission and maintenance therapy. Gastroenterol Hepatol (N Y). 2007;**3**:55-56

[104] Scheinfeld N. Off-label uses and side effects of infliximab. Journal of Drugs in Dermatology. 2004;**3**:273-284

[105] Benitez-del-Castillo JM, Martinez-de-la-Casa JM, Pato-Cour E, Mendez-Fernandez R, Lopez-Abad C, Matilla M, et al. Long-term treatment of refractory posterior uveitis with anti-TNFalpha (infliximab). Eye (London, England). 2005;**19**:841-845

[106] Lopez-Gonzalez R, Loza E, Jover JA, Benitez Del Castillo JM, Mendez R, Hernandez-Garcia C, et al. Treatment of refractory posterior uveitis with infliximab: A 7-year follow-up study. Scandinavian Journal of Rheumatology. 2009;**38**:58-62

[107] Ardoin SP, Kredich D, Rabinovich E, Schanberg LE, Jaffe GJ. Infliximab to treat chronic noninfectious uveitis in children: Retrospective case series with long-term follow-up. American Journal of Ophthalmology. 2007;**144**:844-849

[108] Kahn P, Weiss M, Imundo LF, Levy DM. Favorable response to high-dose infliximab for refractory childhood uveitis. Ophthalmology. 2006;**113**:860-864.e2

[109] Suhler EB, Smith JR, Wertheim MS, Lauer AK, Kurz DE, Pickard TD, et al. A prospective trial of infliximab therapy for refractory uveitis: Preliminary safety and efficacy outcomes. Archives of Ophthalmology. 2005;**123**:903-912

[110] Vallet H, Seve P, Biard L, Baptiste Fraison J, Bielefeld P, Perard L, et al. Infliximab versus adalimumab in the treatment of refractory inflammatory uveitis: A Multicenter Study From the French Uveitis Network. Arthritis & Rhematology. 2016;**68**:1522-1530

[111] Hoshino M, Yoshio T, Onishi S, Minota S. Influence of antibodies against infliximab and etanercept on the treatment effectiveness of these agents in Japanese patients with rheumatoid arthritis. Modern Rheumatology. 2012;**22**:532-540

[112] Napolitano M, Balato N, Ayala F, Cirillo T, Balato A. Multiple sclerosis following anti-tumor necrosis factor-alpha therapy for psoriasis: First case in Italy? Giornale Italiano di Dermatologia e Venereologia. 2018;**153**:567-572

[113] Signore SC, Brauns B, Schutze G, Dohm CP, Bahr M, Mossner R, et al. Infliximab-associated chronic inflammatory central nervous system disease and peroneal nerve injury in a psoriatic patient refractory to treatment: Case report with 10-year follow-up. Case Reports in Neurological Medicine. 2018;**10**:12-17

[114] Remicade. FDA Approved Drug Products [Internet]. 2018. Available from: https://www.accessdata.fda.gov/

drugsatfda_docs/label/2018/103772s5385lbl.pdf

[115] Shealy DJ, Cai A, Staquet K, Baker A, Lacy ER, Johns L, et al. Characterization of golimumab, a human monoclonal antibody specific for human tumor necrosis factor alpha. MAbs. 2010;**2**:428-439

[116] Lowenberg M, de Boer N, Hoentjen F. Golimumab for the treatment of ulcerative colitis. Clinical and Experimental Gastroenterology. 2014;**7**:53-59

[117] Rifkin LM, Birnbaum AD, Goldstein DA. TNF inhibition for ophthalmic indications: Current status and outlook. BioDrugs. 2013;**27**:347-357

[118] Yazgan S, Celik U, Isik M, Yesil NK, Baki AE, Sahin H, et al. Efficacy of golimumab on recurrent uveitis in HLA-B27-positive ankylosing spondylitis. International Ophthalmology. 2017;**37**:139-145

[119] Calvo-Rio V, Blanco R, Santos-Gomez M, Rubio-Romero E, Cordero-Coma M, Gallego-Flores A, et al. Golimumab in refractory uveitis related to spondyloarthritis. Multicenter study of 15 patients. Seminars in Arthritis and Rheumatism. 2016;**46**:95-101

[120] Zhang Z, Fan W, Yang G, Xu Z, Wang J, Cheng Q, et al. Risk of tuberculosis in patients treated with TNF-alpha antagonists: A systematic review and meta-analysis of randomised controlled trials. BMJ Open. 2017;**7**:e012567

[121] Chovel-Sella A, Karplus R, Sella T, Amital H. Clinical efficacy and adverse effects of golimumab in the treatment of rheumatoid arthritis. The Israel Medical Association Journal. 2012;**14**:390-394

[122] Michelon MA, Gottlieb AB. Role of golimumab, a TNF-alpha inhibitor, in the treatment of the psoriatic arthritis. Clinical, Cosmetic and Investigational Dermatology. 2010;**3**:79-84

[123] Duica I, Voinea LM, Mitulescu C, Istrate S, Coman IC, Ciuluvica R. The use of biologic therapies in uveitis. Romanian Journal of Ophthalmology. 2018;**62**:105-113

[124] Simponi. FDA Approved Drug Products [Internet]. 2009. Available from: https://www.accessdata.fda.gov/drugsatfda_docs/label/2009/125289s000lbl.pdf

[125] Lang L. FDA approves Cimzia to treat Crohn's disease. Gastroenterology. 2008;**134**:1819

[126] Llorenc V, Mesquida M, Sainz de la Maza M, Blanco R, Calvo V, Maiz O, et al. Certolizumab Pegol, a New Anti-TNF-alpha in the Armamentarium against Ocular Inflammation. Ocular Immunology and Inflammation. 2016;**24**:167-172

[127] Rudwaleit M, Rosenbaum JT, Landewe R, Marzo-Ortega H, Sieper J, van der Heijde D, et al. Observed incidence of uveitis following certolizumab pegol treatment in patients with axial spondyloarthritis. Arthritis Care & Research (Hoboken). 2016;**68**:838-844

[128] Moisseiev E, Shulman S. Certolizumab-induced uveitis: A case report and review of the literature. Case Reports in Ophthalmology. 2014;**5**:54-59

[129] Acosta-Felquer ML, Rosa J, Soriano ER. An evidence-based review of certolizumab pegol in the treatment of active psoriatic arthritis: Place in therapy. Open Access Rheumatology. 2016;**8**:37-44

[130] Cimzia. FDA Approved Drug Products [Internet]. 2018. Available from: https://www.accessdata.fda.gov/drugsatfda_docs/label/2018/125160s283lbl.pdf

[131] Wan CK, He C, Sun L, Egwuagu CE, Leonard WJ. Cutting edge: IL-1 receptor signaling is critical for the development of autoimmune uveitis. Journal of Immunology. 2016;**196**: 543-546

[132] Lopez-Castejon G, Brough D. Understanding the mechanism of IL-1beta secretion. Cytokine & Growth Factor Reviews. 2011;**22**:189-195

[133] Lin CC, Edelson BT. New insights into the role of IL-1beta in experimental autoimmune encephalomyelitis and multiple sclerosis. Journal of Immunology. 2017;**198**:4553-4560

[134] Sha Y, Markovic-Plese S. A role of IL-1R1 signaling in the differentiation of Th17 cells and the development of autoimmune diseases. Self Nonself. 2011;**2**:35-42

[135] Carreno E, Portero A, Herreras JM, Garcia-Vazquez C, Whitcup SM, Stern ME, et al. Cytokine and chemokine tear levels in patients with uveitis. Acta Ophthalmologica. 2017;**95**:e405-ee14

[136] Arend WP. The balance between IL-1 and IL-1Ra in disease. Cytokine & Growth Factor Reviews. 2002;**13**: 323-340

[137] Goh AX, Bertin-Maghit S, Ping Yeo S, Ho AW, Derks H, Mortellaro A, et al. A novel human anti-interleukin-1beta neutralizing monoclonal antibody showing in vivo efficacy. MAbs. 2014;**6**: 765-773

[138] Dinarello CA, Simon A, van der Meer JW. Treating inflammation by blocking interleukin-1 in a broad spectrum of diseases. Nature Reviews. Drug Discovery. 2012;**11**:633-652

[139] Cohen SB. The use of anakinra, an interleukin-1 receptor antagonist, in the treatment of rheumatoid arthritis. Rheumatic Diseases Clinics of North America. 2004;**30**:365-380, vii

[140] Teoh SC, Sharma S, Hogan A, Lee R, Ramanan AV, Dick AD. Tailoring biological treatment: Anakinra treatment of posterior uveitis associated with the CINCA syndrome. The British Journal of Ophthalmology. 2007;**91**: 263-264

[141] Botsios C, Sfriso P, Ostuni PA, Todesco S, Punzi L. Efficacy of the IL-1 receptor antagonist, anakinra, for the treatment of diffuse anterior scleritis in rheumatoid arthritis. Report of two cases. Rheumatology (Oxford). 2007; **46**:1042-1043

[142] Fabiani C, Vitale A, Emmi G, Lopalco G, Vannozzi L, Guerriero S, et al. Interleukin (IL)-1 inhibition with anakinra and canakinumab in Behcet's disease-related uveitis: A multicenter retrospective observational study. Clinical Rheumatology. 2017;**36**:191-197

[143] Kaiser C, Knight A, Nordstrom D, Pettersson T, Fransson J, Florin-Robertsson E, et al. Injection-site reactions upon Kineret (anakinra) administration: Experiences and explanations. Rheumatology International. 2012;**32**:295-299

[144] Kullenberg T, Lofqvist M, Leinonen M, Goldbach-Mansky R, Olivecrona H. Long-term safety profile of anakinra in patients with severe cryopyrin-associated periodic syndromes. Rheumatology (Oxford). 2016;**55**:1499-1506

[145] Ahmed O, Brahmania M, Alsahafi M, Alkhowaiter S, Erb S. Anakinra hepatotoxicity in a patient with adult-onset still's disease. ACG Case Reports Journal. 2015;**2**:173-174

[146] Fleischmann RM, Tesser J, Schiff MH, Schechtman J, Burmester GR, Bennett R, et al. Safety of extended treatment with anakinra in patients with rheumatoid arthritis. Annals of the Rheumatic Diseases. 2006;**65**:1006-1012

[147] Kineret. FDA Approved Drug Products [Internet]. 2018. Available from: https://www.accessdata.fda.gov/drugsatfda_docs/label/2018/103950s5182lbl.pdf

[148] Dhimolea E. Canakinumab. MAbs. 2010;**2**:3-13

[149] Orrock JE, Ilowite NT. Canakinumab for the treatment of active systemic juvenile idiopathic arthritis. Expert Review of Clinical Pharmacology. 2016;**9**:1015-1024

[150] Hirano M, Seguchi J, Yamamura M, Narita A, Okanobu H, Nishikomori R, et al. Successful resolution of stromal keratitis and uveitis using canakinumab in a patient with chronic infantile neurologic, cutaneous, and articular syndrome: A case study. Journal of Ophthalmic Inflammation and Infection. 2015;**5**:34

[151] Ugurlu S, Ucar D, Seyahi E, Hatemi G, Yurdakul S. Canakinumab in a patient with juvenile Behcet's syndrome with refractory eye disease. Annals of the Rheumatic Diseases. 2012;**71**: 1589-1591

[152] Hoy SM. Canakinumab: A review of its use in the management of systemic juvenile idiopathic arthritis. BioDrugs. 2015;**29**:133-142

[153] Dubois EA, Rissmann R, Cohen AF. Rilonacept and canakinumab. British Journal of Clinical Pharmacology. 2011; **71**:639-641

[154] ILaris. FDA Approved Drug Products [Internet]. 2016. Available from: https://www.accessdata.fda.gov/drugsatfda_docs/label/2016/125319s088lbl.pdf

[155] Knickelbein JE, Tucker WR, Bhatt N, Armbrust K, Valent D, Obiyor D, et al. Gevokizumab in the treatment of autoimmune non-necrotizing anterior scleritis: Results of a phase I/II clinical trial. American Journal of Ophthalmology. 2016;**172**:104-110

[156] Gul A, Tugal-Tutkun I, Dinarello CA, Reznikov L, Esen BA, Mirza A, et al. Interleukin-1beta-regulating antibody XOMA 052 (gevokizumab) in the treatment of acute exacerbations of resistant uveitis of Behcet's disease: An open-label pilot study. Annals of the Rheumatic Diseases. 2012;**71**:563-566

[157] Tugal-Tutkun IM, Kadayifcilar SM, Khairallah MM, Lee SCMP, Ozdal P, Ozyazgan Y, et al. Safety and efficacy of gevokizumab in patients with Behcet's disease uveitis: Results of an exploratory phase 2 study. Ocular Immunology and Inflammation. 2017;**25**:62-70

[158] Tugal-Tutkun I, Pavesio C, De Cordoue A, Bernard-Poenaru O, Gul A. Use of gevokizumab in patients with Behcet's disease uveitis: An international, randomized, double-masked, placebo-controlled study and open-label extension study. Ocular Immunology and Inflammation. 2018:1-11

[159] Cavelti-Weder C, Babians-Brunner A, Keller C, Stahel MA, Kurz-Levin M, Zayed H, et al. Effects of gevokizumab on glycemia and inflammatory markers in typ. 2 diabetes. Diabetes Care. 2012; **35**:1654-1662

[160] Kapur S, Bonk ME. Rilonacept (arcalyst), an interleukin-1 trap for the treatment of cryopyrin-associated periodic syndromes. P T. 2009;**34**: 138-141

[161] Gomes Bittencourt M, Sepah YJ, Do DV, Agbedia O, Akhtar A, Liu H, et al. New treatment options for noninfectious uveitis. Developments in Ophthalmology. 2012;**51**:134-161

[162] Gillespie J, Mathews R, McDermott MF. Rilonacept in the management of cryopyrin-associated periodic syndromes (CAPS). Journal of Inflammation Research. 2010;**3**:1-8

[163] Vitale A, Rigante D, Lucherini OM, Caso F, Muscari I, Magnotti F, et al. Biological treatments: New weapons in the management of monogenic autoinflammatory disorders. Mediators of Inflammation. 2013;**2013**:939847

[164] Arcalyst. FDA Approved Drug Products [Internet]. 2008. Available from: https://www.accessdata.fda.gov/drugsatfda_docs/label/2008/125249lbl.pdf

[165] Maccio A, Madeddu C. The role of interleukin-6 in the evolution of ovarian cancer: Clinical and prognostic implications–A review. Journal of Molecular Medicine (Berlin). 2013;**91**:1355-1368

[166] Grevich S, Shenoi S. Update on the management of systemic juvenile idiopathic arthritis and role of IL-1 and IL-6 inhibition. Adolescent Health, Medicine and Therapeutics. 2017;**8**:125-135

[167] Tappeiner C, Heinz C, Ganser G, Heiligenhaus A. Is tocilizumab an effective option for treatment of refractory uveitis associated with juvenile idiopathic arthritis? The Journal of Rheumatology. 2012;**39**:1294-1295

[168] Adan A, Mesquida M, Llorenc V, Espinosa G, Molins B, Hernandez MV, et al. Tocilizumab treatment for refractory uveitis-related cystoid macular edema. Graefe's Archive for Clinical and Experimental Ophthalmology. 2013;**251**:2627-2632

[169] Tappeiner C, Mesquida M, Adan A, Anton J, Ramanan AV, Carreno E, et al. Evidence for tocilizumab as a treatment option in refractory uveitis associated with juvenile idiopathic arthritis. The Journal of Rheumatology. 2016;**43**:2183-2188

[170] Sepah YJ, Sadiq MA, Chu DS, Dacey M, Gallemore R, Dayani P, et al. Primary (month-6) outcomes of the STOP-uveitis study: Evaluating the safety, tolerability, and efficacy of tocilizumab in patients with noninfectious uveitis. American Journal of Ophthalmology. 2017;**183**:71-80

[171] Chen J, Chen S, He J. A case of refractory intestinal Behcet's disease treated with tocilizumab, a humanised anti-interleukin-6 receptor antibody. 2017. Clinical and Experimental Rheumatology;**108**(35 Suppl):116-118

[172] Oshitari T, Kajita F, Tobe A, Itami M, Yotsukura J, Baba T, et al. Refractory uveitis in patient with castleman disease successfully treated with tocilizumab. Case Reports in Ophthalmological Medicine. 2012;**2012**:968180

[173] Ruiz-Medrano J, Diaz-Valle D, Cuina R, Gegundez JA, Chhablani J, Majumder PD, et al. The role of tocilizumab in the treatment of inflammatory diseases of the eye and orbit: A useful alternative. Journal Français d'Ophtalmologie. 2018;**8**:759-766

[174] Jones G, Ding C. Tocilizumab: A review of its safety and efficacy in rheumatoid arthritis. Clinical Medicine Insights: Arthritis and Musculoskeletal Disorders. 2010;**3**:81-89

[175] Monemi S, Berber E, Sarsour K, Wang J, Lampl K, Bharucha K, et al. Incidence of gastrointestinal perforations in patients with rheumatoid arthritis treated with tocilizumab from clinical trial, postmarketing, and real-world data sources. Rheumatology and Theraphy. 2016;**3**:337-352

[176] Xie F, Yun H, Bernatsky S, Curtis JR. Brief report: Risk of gastrointestinal perforation among rheumatoid arthritis patients receiving tofacitinib, tocilizumab, or other biologic

treatments. Arthritis & Rhematology. 2016;**68**:2612-2617

[177] Rubbert-Roth A, Sebba A, Brockwell L, Kelman A, Porter-Brown B, Pulley J, et al. Malignancy rates in patients with rheumatoid arthritis treated with tocilizumab. RMD Open. 2016;**2**:e000213

[178] Actemra. FDA Approved Drug Products [Internet]. 2018. Available from: https://www.accessdata.fda.gov/drugsatfda_docs/label/2018/125276s122,125472s031lbl.pdf

[179] Takayanagi N. Biological agents and respiratory infections: Causative mechanisms and practice management. Respiratory Investigation. 2015;**53**:185-200

[180] McCarty D, Robinson A. Efficacy and safety of sarilumab in patients with active rheumatoid arthritis. Therapeutic Advances in Musculoskeletal Disease. 2018;**10**:61-67

[181] Maya JR, Sadiq MA, Zapata LJ, Hanout M, Sarwar S, Rajagopalan N, et al. Emerging therapies for noninfectious uveitis: What may be coming to the clinics. Journal of Ophthalmology. 2014;**2014**:310329

[182] Boyce EG, Rogan EL, Vyas D, Prasad N, Mai Y. Sarilumab: Review of a second IL-6 receptor antagonist indicated for the treatment of rheumatoid arthritis. The Annals of Pharmacotherapy. 2018;**52**:780-791

[183] Kevzara. FDA Approved Drug Products [Internet]. 2018. Available from: https://www.accessdata.fda.gov/drugsatfda_docs/label/2018/761037s001lbl.pdf

[184] Mease P, Strand V, Shalamberidze L, Dimic A, Raskina T, Xu LA, et al. A phase II, double-blind, randomised, placebo-controlled study of BMS945429 (ALD518) in patients with rheumatoid arthritis with an inadequate response to methotrexate. Annals of the Rheumatic Diseases. 2012;**71**:1183-1189

[185] Genovese MC, Fleischmann R, Furst D, Janssen N, Carter J, Dasgupta B, et al. Efficacy and safety of olokizumab in patients with rheumatoid arthritis with an inadequate response to TNF inhibitor therapy: Outcomes of a randomised Phase IIb study. Annals of the Rheumatic Diseases. 2014;**73**:1607-1615

[186] Smolen JS, Weinblatt ME, Sheng S, Zhuang Y, Hsu B. Sirukumab, a human anti-interleukin-6 monoclonal antibody: A randomised, 2-part (proof-of-concept and dose-finding), phase II study in patients with active rheumatoid arthritis despite methotrexate therapy. Annals of the Rheumatic Diseases. 2014;**73**:1616-1625

[187] Kurzrock R, Voorhees PM, Casper C, Furman RR, Fayad L, Lonial S, et al. A phase I, open-label study of siltuximab, an anti-IL-6 monoclonal antibody, in patients with B-cell non-Hodgkin lymphoma, multiple myeloma, or Castleman disease. Clinical Cancer Research. 2013;**19**:3659-3670

[188] Correction to Lancet HIV 2017. Lancet HIV. 2017;**4**:e122-e133. 4: e102

[189] Veldhoen M. Interleukin 17 is a chief orchestrator of immunity. Nature Immunology. 2017;**18**:612-621

[190] Guedes MC, Borrego LM, Proenca RD. Roles of interleukin-17 in uveitis. Indian Journal of Ophthalmology. 2016;**64**:628-634

[191] Kellner H. Targeting interleukin-17 in patients with active rheumatoid arthritis: Rationale and clinical potential. Therapeutic Advances in Musculoskeletal Disease. 2013;**5**:141-152

[192] Kunwar S, Dahal K, Sharma S. Anti-IL-17 therapy in treatment of rheumatoid arthritis: A systematic literature review and meta-analysis of randomized controlled trials. Rheumatology International. 2016;**36**: 1065-1075

[193] Thomas LW, Lee EB, Wu JJ. Systematic review of anti-drug antibodies of IL-17 inhibitors for psoriasis. The Journal of Dermatological Treatment. 2018:1-7

[194] Luger D, Silver PB, Tang J, Cua D, Chen Z, Iwakura Y, et al. Either a Th17 or a Th1 effector response can drive autoimmunity: Conditions of disease induction affect dominant effector category. The Journal of Experimental Medicine. 2008;**205**:799-810

[195] Fala L. Cosentyx (Secukinumab): First IL-17A antagonist receives FDA approval for moderate-to-severe plaque psoriasis. American Health & Drug Benefits. 2016;**9**:60-63

[196] Hueber W, Patel DD, Dryja T, Wright AM, Koroleva I, Bruin G, et al. Effects of AIN457, a fully human antibody to interleukin-17A, on psoriasis, rheumatoid arthritis, and uveitis. Science Translational Medicine. 2010;**2**:52ra72

[197] Dick AD, Tugal-Tutkun I, Foster S, Zierhut M, Melissa Liew SH, Bezlyak V, et al. Secukinumab in the treatment of noninfectious uveitis: Results of three randomized, controlled clinical trials. Ophthalmology. 2013;**120**:777-787

[198] Letko E, Yeh S, Foster CS, Pleyer U, Brigell M, Grosskreutz CL, et al. Efficacy and safety of intravenous secukinumab in noninfectious uveitis requiring steroid-sparing immunosuppressive therapy. Ophthalmology. 2015;**122**:939-948

[199] Fobelo Lozano MJ, Serrano Gimenez R, Castro Fernandez M. Emergence of inflammatory bowel disease during treatment with secukinumab. Journal of Crohn's & Colitis. 2018;**12**:1131-1133

[200] Frieder J, Kivelevitch D, Menter A. Secukinumab: A review of the anti-IL-17A biologic for the treatment of psoriasis. Therapeutic Advances in Chronic Disease. 2018;**9**:5-21

[201] Cosentyx. FDA Approved Drug Products [Internet]. 2018. Available from: https://www.accessdata.fda.gov/drugsatfda_docs/label/2018/125504s013lbl.pdf

[202] Kammuller M, Tsai TF, Griffiths CE, Kapoor N, Kolattukudy PE, Brees D, et al. Inhibition of IL-17A by secukinumab shows no evidence of increased Mycobacterium tuberculosis infections. Clinical & Translational Immunology. 2017;**6**:e152

[203] Blauvelt A. Safety of secukinumab in the treatment of psoriasis. Expert Opinion on Drug Safety. 2016;**15**: 1413-1420

[204] Butler NJ, Suhler EB, Rosenbaum JT. Interferon alpha 2b in the treatment of uveitic cystoid macular edema. Ocular Immunology and Inflammation. 2012;**20**:86-90

[205] Kivity S, Katz U, Daniel N, Nussinovitch U, Papageorgiou N, Shoenfeld Y. Evidence for the use of intravenous immunoglobulins–A review of the literature. Clinical Reviews in Allergy and Immunology. 2010;**38**: 201-269

[206] Garcia-Geremias M, Carreno E, Epps SJ, Lee RW, Dick AD. Clinical outcomes of intravenous immunoglobulin therapy in refractory uveitis. International Ophthalmology. 2015;**35**:281-285

[207] You C, Lamba N, Lasave AF, Ma L, Diaz MH, Foster CS. Rituximab in the treatment of ocular cicatricial pemphigoid: A retrospective cohort study. Graefe's Archive for Clinical and Experimental Ophthalmology. 2017;**255**: 1221-1228

[208] Ahmed A, Foster CS. Cyclophosphamide or rituximab treatment of scleritis and uveitis for patients with granulomatosis with polyangiitis. Ophthalmic Research. 2018. DOI: 10.1159/000486791

[209] Reynolds A, Koenig AS, Bananis E, Singh A. When is switching warranted among biologic therapies in rheumatoid arthritis? Expert Review of Pharmacoeconomics & Outcomes Research. 2012;**12**:319-333

[210] Wei W, Knapp K, Wang L, Chen CI, Craig GL, Ferguson K, et al. Treatment persistence and clinical outcomes of tumor necrosis factor inhibitor cycling or switching to a new mechanism of action therapy: Real-world observational study of rheumatoid arthritis patients in the United States with prior tumor necrosis factor inhibitor therapy. Advances in Therapy. 2017;**34**:1936-1952

[211] Kraus CL, Culican SM. Use of biologic agents in ocular manifestations of rheumatic disease. International Journal of Clinical Rheumatology. 2012; **2012**:203819

Chapter 8

# Tumor Necrosis Factor-Alpha Inhibitory Therapy for Non-Infectious Autoimmune Uveitis

*Judy L. Chen, Ann-Marie Lobo-Chan, Robison Vernon Paul Chan and Pooja Bhat*

## Abstract

Biologic agents represent a mainstay in the treatment of refractory non-infectious, immune-mediated uveitis. Tumor necrosis factor (TNF)-α inhibitors have demonstrated efficacy in inducing and sustaining disease remission in numerous systemic inflammatory disorders and their associated uveitic entities. In particular, studies have shown that infliximab and adalimumab can induce steroid-free disease remission in patients with Behçet's disease and juvenile arthritis as treatments that are superior to conventional disease-modifying immunosuppressive agents. Patients receiving anti-TNF-α therapy may experience adverse events and should be closely monitored for the development of opportunistic infections, reactivation of tuberculosis and hepatitis, demyelinating disease and neuropathies, as well as malignancies.

**Keywords:** TNF-alpha inhibitors, uveitis, ocular inflammation, etanercept, infliximab, adalimumab, golimumab, certolizumab

## 1. Introduction and overview

- *Mechanism of action*: TNF-α inhibitors suppress the robust systemic and ocular inflammatory response triggered by tumor necrosis factor.

- *Formulations & application to uveitis*: the currently available agents include etanercept, a TNF receptor fusion protein that binds TNF-α and TNF-β, as well as monoclonal antibodies infliximab, adalimumab, golimumab, and certolizumab that bind and neutralize soluble and transmembrane TNF. TNF-α inhibitors have been used efficaciously in uveitis associated with systemic disease, most notably Behçet's disease and juvenile idiopathic arthritis, as well as idiopathic intermediate, posterior and panuveitis.

- *Adverse effects*: important side effects of TNF-α inhibitors include malignancy (lymphomas, skin cancer), infections (reactivation of latent tuberculosis and hepatitis, fungal and various opportunistic infections), demyelinating disease, congestive heart failure, induction of auto-antibodies, and injection site reactions.

- *Monitoring clinical response and serum anti-drug antibodies*: a major concern in patients who demonstrate suboptimal response or fail anti-TNF-α therapy is the development of drug antibodies, which may warrant switching agents to either another TNF antagonist, or alternative immunosuppression.

## 2. Mechanism of action

### 2.1 Physiology of TNF

Tumor necrosis factors are pro-inflammatory cytokines that play an integral role in innate and adaptive immunity. These factors exist in two forms as TNF-α and TNF-β (or lymphotoxin), and were named for *in vitro* observations of their induction of tumor cell lysis and necrosis [1]. Also referred to as sentinel cytokines or "the body's fire alarm," TNFs have since been discovered to initiate the host defense response to local injury and infections, notably those caused by mycobacterial, fungal, and other opportunistic pathogens. TNFs are also responsible for formation of lymphoid tissue, as well as activation and recruitment of leukocytes, including neutrophils and macrophages for granuloma formation [2]. The physiologic functions of TNF explain many of the adverse effects associated with TNF blockade, including cytopenias; increased risk for infection, particularly reactivation of hepatitis and tuberculosis; as well as higher incidence of certain malignancies, discussed in more detail later in this chapter. Regulation of TNF is intricate, and encompasses a variety

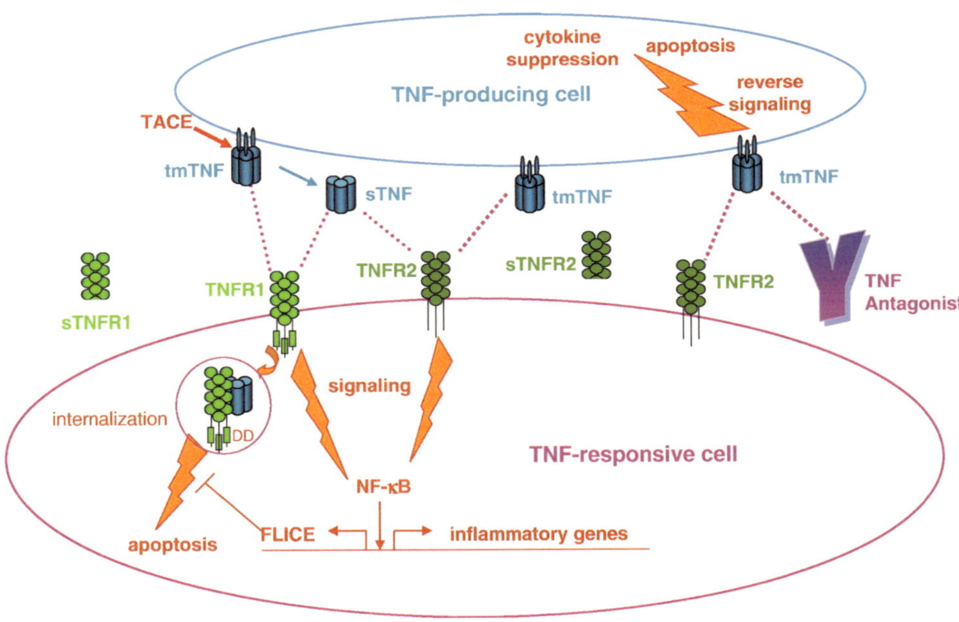


**Figure 1.**
*TNF production, receptor interaction, and signaling (taken with permission from Tracey et al. [2]). Stimulation of a TNF-producing cell (top) results in cell surface expression of tmTNF trimers and enzymatic cleavage by TACE to release sTNF. Both tmTNF and sTNF can bind to cell surface TNFR1 or TNFR2 on a TNF-responsive cell (bottom), initiating signaling pathways that lead to apoptosis or NF-κB activation and inflammatory gene activation. The induction of apoptosis by sTNF via TNFR1 involves internalization of the ligand-receptor complex and association of death domains (DD) in the cytoplasmic tail of TNFR1 with adapter proteins and is normally blocked by FADD-like IL-1β–converting enzyme (FLICE). Reverse signaling can be initiated by TNFR2 or TNF antagonist binding to cell surface tmTNF, resulting in cytokine suppression or apoptosis. Soluble TNF receptors (sTNFR1 and sTNFR2) can be released from a TNF-responsive cell following enzymatic cleavage. TNF antagonists bind sTNF and tmTNF to neutralize their effects. TACE = tumor necrosis factor-alpha converting enzyme; NF-κβ = nuclear factor kappa β.*

of stimuli, TNF-producing and responsive cells, and feedback loops. Numerous immune cells, including activated macrophages, T cells, mast cells, granulocytes, and natural killer cells, produce TNF in the form of transmembrane TNF (tmTNF) and soluble TNF (sTNF), which is cleaved from tmTNF (**Figure 1**). Initial production of these factors may be triggered by a wide array of stimuli, including microbial pathogens, tumor cells, immune complexes, other cytokines, complement factors, irradiation, ischemia or hypoxia, and trauma [2].

Ultimately, both tmTNF and sTNF act upon TNF-responsive cells to trigger an inflammatory response via membrane-bound TNF receptors 1 and 2 (TNFR1 and TNFR2). TNFR1, also known as p55, is constitutively expressed on nearly all cell types except erythrocytes. Depending on the metabolic state of the cell, binding of TNFR1 triggers one of two distinct signaling pathways: (1) activation of nuclear factor kappa-β, a family of transcription factors that controls many inflammatory genes, or (2) caspase-dependent apoptosis [2]. TNFR2, also known as p75, is preferentially expressed on endothelial and hematopoietic cells, and some tumor cells. The subsequent pathways at this time are not as well delineated as those for TNFR1, but ongoing studies suggest TNFR2 mediates the activity of regulatory and effector CD8+ T cells, as well as interleukin production by B cells [3, 4]. In the eye, pigment epithelial cells of the iris, the ciliary body, and retina locally express TNFR1 and TNFR2.

Positive and negative feedback loops initiated by TNF-induced factors regulate TNF production. Proteolytic cleavage of the extracellular domain of membrane-bound TNF receptors results in soluble TNF receptors, which bind and neutralize

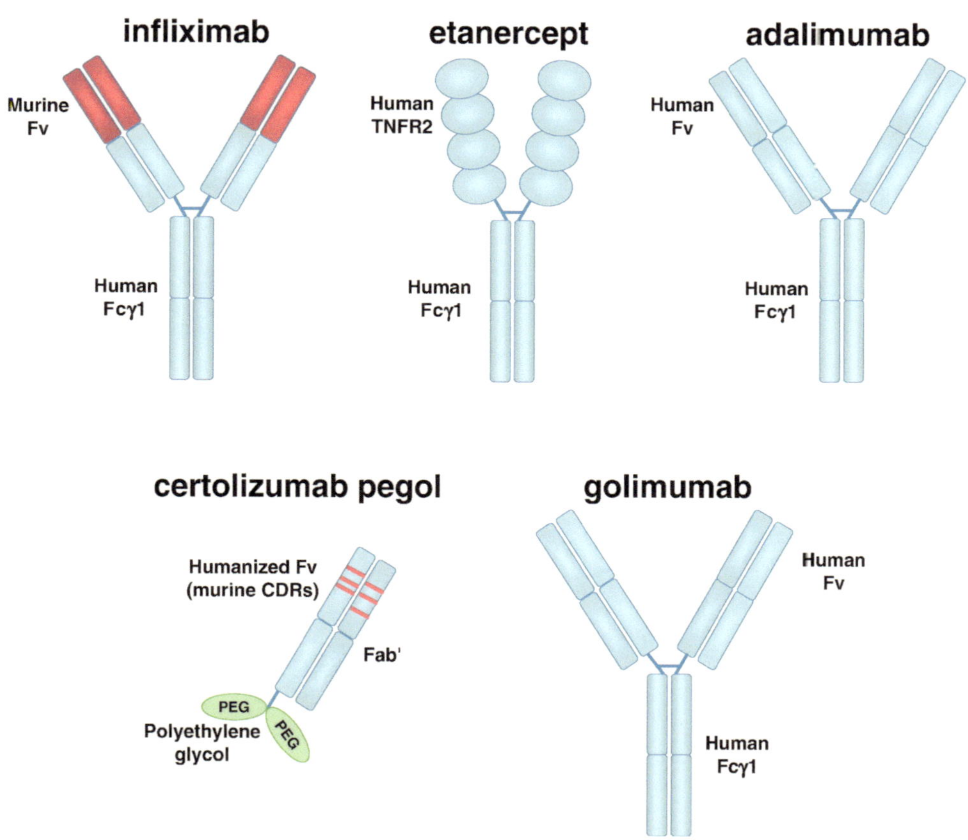


**Figure 2.**
*Downstream effects of TNF depicting the common cascades leading to immune regulation, apoptosis, and inflammation (center), as well as biologic activities specific to the pathophysiology of Crohn's disease, rheumatoid arthritis, and psoriasis (taken with permission from Tracey et al. [2]).*

TNF without inciting inflammation [5]. This maintains the amount of circulating TNF below pathologic limits, and thus healthy individuals do not typically express detectable serum levels of these factors.

## 2.2 TNF blockade

In immune-mediated disease, high concentrations of TNF induce excessive systemic inflammation and organ injury via direct pathogenic effects and production of other inflammatory mediators, apoptosis, and tissue destruction (**Figure 2**). TNF-α has been implicated in the pathogenesis of not only uveitis, but also commonly associated complications of ocular inflammation, including cystoid macular edema and choroidal neovascularization. Increased expression and production of TNF-α has been found to be crucial in the induction phase of experimental autoimmune uveitis, and inhibition of TNF-α in these experimental models of uveitis reduces the incidence and severity of intraocular inflammation [6].

Given the key role of TNF as a mediator of inflammation, its potential as a pharmaceutical target for blockade has been recognized, and several agents that antagonize TNF and TNF receptors have been created. Etanercept, the sole inhibitor in its class that is not a monoclonal antibody, is a soluble dimeric fusion protein

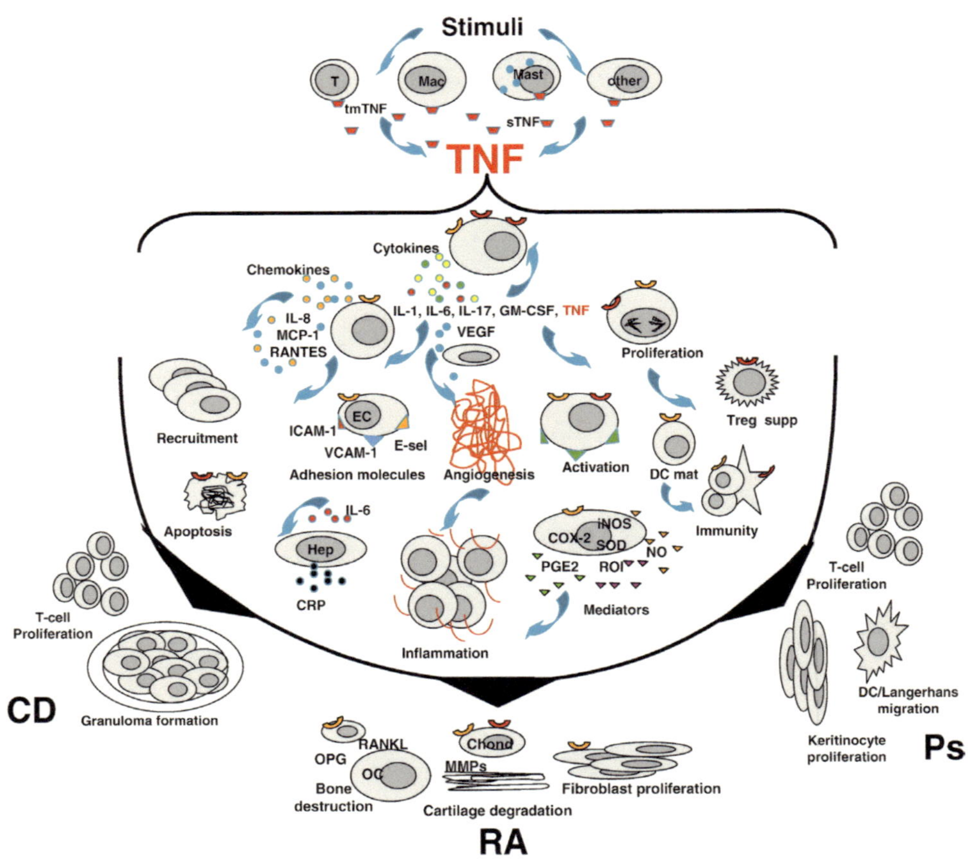


**Figure 3.**
*Molecular structures of the available TNF inhibitors (taken with permission from Tracey et al. [2]). Infliximab is a mouse/human chimeric monoclonal anti-TNF antibody of IgG1 isotype. Adalimumab and golimumab are fully human IgG1 monoclonal anti-TNF antibodies. Etanercept is a fusion protein of TNFR2 (p75) and the Fc region of human IgG1. Certolizumab is a PEGylated Fab' fragment of a humanized IgG1 monoclonal anti-TNF antibody. Fv = variable fragment domain; Fcγ1 = crystallizable fragment domain of IgG1; CDR = complementarity determining region.*

that carries two copies of the ligand-binding portion of the TNF receptor p75 linked to the crystallizable fragment (Fc) region of human immunoglobulin G (IgG). This forms unstable complexes with and transiently neutralizes both TNF-α and TNF-β, in contrast to the other agents that bind only TNF-α.

The remainder of this class comprises monoclonal antibodies that bind both sTNF and tmTNF, with certain structural variations between agents (**Figure 3**). Infliximab is a chimeric mouse-human monoclonal antibody, with murine fragment antigen-binding regions (Fab) that bind soluble and bound TNF-α to inactivate them. Adalimumab and golimumab, on the other hand, also bind soluble and transmembrane forms of TNF-α, but are fully human; the absence of non-human components renders them less immunogenic and, therefore, less subject to the formation of anti-drug antibodies as compared to infliximab. Similarly, certolizumab pegol is humanized, but is also distinct from the others in that this compound couples the Fab region to polyethylene glycol rather than the Fc region of human IgG. This reduces the antigenicity of this agent and increases the half-life of the drug [7]. The absence of the Fc portion of human IgG also precludes the typical antibody effector functions of complement activation, apoptosis induction, and neutrophil degranulation [2]. Further information regarding each of these agents is detailed in the section below.

## 3. Formulations and their application to uveitis

Currently, TNF inhibitors are approved by the United States Food and Drug Administration (FDA) for use in many immune-mediated conditions, including rheumatoid arthritis, juvenile arthritis, ankylosing spondylitis, inflammatory bowel disease, and psoriasis and psoriatic arthritis. Only adalimumab has been approved currently by the FDA for non-infectious intermediate, posterior and panuveitis in adults and children older than 2 years of age. Though their use for uveitis is considered off-label, the remaining anti-TNF agents have been routinely used to control ocular inflammation associated with systemic disease. These medications have been found to be particularly effective in Behçet's disease and juvenile idiopathic arthritis, as well as intermediate, posterior, and panuveitis of idiopathic and other causes. In general, initial response to TNF-α inhibitors is more rapid than other immunomodulatory agents, which can take several weeks to months to become therapeutic. Recommendations regarding administration and dosing of these agents are not specific to the treatment of uveitis, but are derived from rheumatologic literature. **Table 1** summarizes the available TNF antagonists.

### 3.1 Etanercept

Etanercept (Enbrel®, Amgen Wyeth, Immunex Corporation, Thousand Oaks, CA, USA) was the first anti-TNF-α agent to be approved by the FDA in 1998 for use in rheumatoid arthritis, polyarticular juvenile idiopathic arthritis, ankylosing spondylitis, psoriatic arthritis, and plaque psoriasis. The compound consists of a humanized, recombinant dimeric fusion of a human Fc molecule and two p75 TNF receptors. By binding circulating TNF-α and TNF-β, etanercept prevents binding of these factors to cell surface TNF receptors and the subsequent pro-inflammatory cascade. Of note, unlike other agents within its class, etanercept does not bind tmTNF, and thus does not induce lysis of TNF-producing cells.

#### *3.1.1 Administration*

Etanercept is administered as subcutaneous injections dosed 50 mg once weekly or 25 mg twice weekly. Higher doses may be used short term in some conditions.

| | Etanercept (Enbrel) | Infliximab (Remicade) | Adalimumab (Humira) | Golimumab (Simponi, Simponi Aria) | Certolizumab (Cimzia) |
|---|---|---|---|---|---|
| Structure and mechanism of action | Dimeric fusion protein of TNF receptors that binds TNF-α and TNF-β | Chimeric mouse-human monoclonal antibody that binds TNF-α | Fully humanized monoclonal antibody that binds TNF-α | Fully humanized monoclonal antibody that binds TNF-α | PEGylated antigen-binding fragment that binds TNF-α |
| Route of administration and dosages | Subcutaneous injection (50 mg weekly or 25 mg twice weekly) | Intravenous infusion (loading: 3–5 mg/kg at 0, 2, and 6 weeks; maintenance: 3–10 mg/kg monthly every 4–8 weeks, up to 20 mg/kg monthly in children) | Subcutaneous injection (80 mg loading dose, followed by 40 mg every 1–2 weeks) | Subcutaneous injection (50 mg monthly) or intravenous infusion (loading: 2 mg/kg at weeks 0 and 4; maintenance: every 8 weeks) | Subcutaneous injection (loading: 400 mg at weeks 0, 2, and 4; maintenance: 400 mg injections monthly, or 200 mg injections every other week) |
| Approved indications | Rheumatoid arthritis, juvenile idiopathic arthritis, psoriatic arthritis, ankylosing spondylitis | Rheumatoid arthritis, ankylosing spondylitis, psoriatic arthritis, Crohn's disease, ulcerative colitis | Noninfectious intermediate, posterior and panuveitis; rheumatoid arthritis, juvenile idiopathic arthritis, psoriatic arthritis, ankylosing spondylitis, Crohn's disease, ulcerative colitis | Rheumatoid arthritis, ankylosing spondylitis, psoriatic arthritis | Rheumatoid arthritis |
| Adverse events | Opportunistic and invasive fungal infections, reactivation of underlying hepatitis and tuberculosis infections, malignancies (lymphoma, skin cancers), demyelinating disease, congestive heart failure, induction of autoimmunity | | | | |

**Table 1.**
*Summary of the available TNF inhibitors, their structures and mechanisms of action, routes and dosages of administration, and adverse effects.*

### 3.1.2 Efficacy

Etanercept appears to be inferior to infliximab and adalimumab for the control of ocular inflammation and is generally considered inadequate for the treatment of uveitis [8]. It should be noted that the present data are mostly small series, and no large, prospective head-to-head studies exist comparing effectiveness or safety across the TNF-α antagonists. However, use of etanercept has consistently shown decreased initial response, greater corticosteroid burden, and higher rates of disease recurrence than have been reported with the use of infliximab for uveitis [9]. Furthermore, etanercept has been associated with the paradoxical development of *de novo* uveitis and induction of uveitis flares in patients with spondyloarthropathies, rheumatoid arthritis, juvenile idiopathic arthritis, and sarcoidosis [10]. The mechanism for this is unclear, but is thought to be related to pharmacokinetic differences between etanercept and other TNF inhibitors, or differences in reverse signaling, such as cytokine modulation [2].

#### *3.1.3 Safety*

A recent prospective analysis of etanercept, infliximab, and adalimumab found that the rate of infection requiring hospitalization, intravenous antibiotics, or life-threatening complications or disability is lower with etanercept than with infliximab or adalimumab [11].

### 3.2 Infliximab

Infliximab (Remicade®, Janssen Biotech, Inc., Horsham, PA, USA) was the second anti-TNF-α agent to receive FDA approval in 1999 for treatment of rheumatoid arthritis, ulcerative colitis, Crohn's disease, ankylosing spondylitis, psoriatic arthritis, and plaque psoriasis. This drug is a chimeric mouse-human monoclonal antibody that binds and neutralizes both circulating and membrane-bound TNF-α.

#### *3.2.1 Administration*

Infliximab is only available as an intravenous infusion. Typical loading regimens involve initial doses of 3–5 mg/kg at 0, 2, and 6 weeks, though the loading dosages may vary based on disease etiology and severity. Once a steady state has been achieved following the loading period, patients undergo regular infusions approximately every 4–8 weeks. Maintenance doses may be safely increased to 5–10 mg/kg monthly, though in JIA, children may require higher doses (up to 20 mg/kg) to successfully quell disease [12].

#### *3.2.2 Efficacy*

Numerous studies have established the efficacy of infliximab in various etiologies of uveitis, with the most data supporting its use in Behçet's disease and juvenile idiopathic arthritis. Consistently, infliximab is associated with a decrease in the mean corticosteroid dose and immunosuppression load required for management of ocular inflammation. Patients with Behçet's disease-related uveitis and retinal vasculitis have been shown to achieve faster resolution of disease with infliximab than with local and systemic corticosteroid therapy, or other immunomodulatory agents [13, 14]. Markomichelakis et al. performed a prospective, observational study of patients with panuveitis secondary to Behçet's disease who received a single dose of infliximab infusion of 5 mg/kg, high-dose methylprednisolone 1 g/day for 3 days, or intravitreal triamcinolone; infliximab was found to be superior to other treatments in terms of decreasing ocular inflammation, and clearing retinal vasculitis, retinitis, and cystoid macular edema [13]. Many children with JIA and chronic refractory noninfectious uveitis also achieve improvement as well as quiescence of disease with the addition of infliximab to methotrexate [15]. A review of 16 children on concomitant infliximab (mean dose 8.2 mg/kg with a median interval of 5.6 weeks between infusions) and methotrexate therapy found that this regimen effectively controlled ocular inflammation over 1 year of follow-up, without recurrence of uveitis in 58% of patients [15]. Reports also suggest efficacy of infliximab in the treatment of uveitis related to many other conditions, including spondyloarthropathies, inflammatory bowel disease, psoriasis, Takayasu disease, pars planitis, multifocal choroiditis, birdshot chorioretinopathy, Vogt-Koyanagi-Harada syndrome, sympathetic ophthalmia, and idiopathic uveitis. Infliximab use has also shown benefit in recalcitrant uveitic cystoid macular edema and diffuse subretinal fibrosis [16, 17]. In a study of nine patients with uveitis-related cystoid macular edema refractory to conventional immunosuppressive therapy, Schaap-Fogler et al. reported that after transitioning to infliximab (dosage of 5 mg/kg at 0, 2, and 6 weeks, followed by administration every 6–8 weeks afterward) or adalimumab (dosage of 40 mg every 2 weeks), patients experienced improvement in central macular thickness and visual acuities comparable to those on conventional immunomodulatory therapy on follow-up at 3, 6, and 12 months [16].

In a small percentage of patients, the formation of human anti-chimeric antibodies, or HACA, may neutralize infliximab and limit its duration of effect. Other immunomodulatory agents may be administered concurrently with infliximab to reduce the rate of HACA formation. Further discussion regarding the development of HACA and approach to patients who have failed therapy is detailed in the section "Adverse effects."

#### *3.2.3 Safety*

Infliximab has been associated with significant adverse effects, including serious infections, congestive heart failure, pulmonary embolus, induction of autoantibodies, as well as development of a rare lupus-like syndrome [11, 18].

### 3.3 Adalimumab

Adalimumab (Humira®, AbbVie Inc., North Chicago, IL, USA) is a fully humanized monoclonal antibody against TNF-α. Since its approval by the FDA in 2002, it has been steadily gaining popularity for its efficacy and relative safety, and now serves as a preferred agent within its class. At this time, its approved indications include treatment of rheumatoid arthritis, ulcerative colitis, Crohn's disease, psoriatic arthritis, plaque psoriasis, ankylosing spondylitis, and juvenile idiopathic arthritis. In 2016, it was approved by the FDA for treatment of non-infectious intermediate, posterior and panuveitis.

#### *3.3.1 Administration*

Adalimumab is delivered in the form of subcutaneous injections with a loading dose of 80 mg followed by 40 mg injections at weekly or biweekly intervals.

#### *3.3.2 Efficacy*

Numerous studies have shown adalimumab to be efficacious, particularly in uveitis associated with spondyloarthropathies, HLA-B27 positive status, and juvenile idiopathic arthritis. There also exists moderate-quality evidence for the efficacy of adalimumab in Behçet's disease-associated uveitis, pars planitis, and idiopathic posterior uveitis. A multinational randomized controlled trial evaluating adalimumab for the treatment of active noninfectious intermediate, posterior, or panuveitis despite prednisone therapy revealed significant improvement in anterior and posterior chamber inflammation as well as visual acuity [19]. Compared to placebo, adalimumab achieved early and sustained disease control after discontinuation of glucocorticoid treatment, with less chance of treatment failure and increased median time to treatment failure (24 weeks in adalimumab group versus 13 weeks in placebo group) [19]. Like infliximab, adalimumab allows for a significant reduction in the mean corticosteroid dose and mean immunosuppression load required in noninfectious uveitis. Furthermore, adalimumab has been associated with improvement in uveitic macular edema in prospective trials, which may be related to a reduction in plasma anti-VEGF levels with therapy [20].

Though less immunogenic than infliximab, adalimumab may still induce the formation of anti-drug antibodies in some patients, which may neutralize and limit the efficacy of the drug over time.

#### *3.3.3 Safety*

Overall, adalimumab is relatively safe for patients, and it is uncommon that the drug induces adverse events necessitating its discontinuation. Rates of lupus-like syndromes, and demyelinating disease and neuropathies, including optic neuritis, have been reportedly lower as compared to infliximab and etanercept. However, use of adalimumab still carries the risk of potentially devastating infections, including respiratory tract infections and reactivation of tuberculosis.

### 3.4 Golimumab

Golimumab (Simponi® and Simponi Aria®, Janssen Biotech, Inc., Horsham, PA, USA) was approved by the FDA in 2009 for the treatment of moderate to severe active rheumatoid arthritis, psoriatic arthritis, ankylosing spondylitis, and ulcerative colitis. Like adalimumab, golimumab is a fully human monoclonal antibody.

#### *3.4.1 Administration*

Golimumab is delivered either as monthly subcutaneous injections of 50 mg each month or as intravenous infusions. Similar to infliximab, the intravenous form of golimumab is loaded at 2 mg/kg at weeks 0 and 4 and then maintained with infusions every 8 weeks.

#### *3.4.2 Efficacy*

A limited number of case series describe success in treating cases of uveitis associated with ankylosing spondylitis, HLA-B27 positive status, juvenile idiopathic arthritis, and Behçet's disease after inadequate response to or intolerance of other TNF-α inhibitors [21, 22]. In a 2014 study by Miserocchi et al. of 17 affected patients, 14 patients experienced improvement in inflammation with golimumab therapy, with the majority achieving quiescence and corticosteroid-sparing effect over an average follow-up of 21.9 months [21]. Of note, the remaining three subjects were deemed non-responders.

#### *3.4.3 Safety*

Existing reports on the use of golimumab have not reported a significantly different rate of adverse events compared to that for other TNF inhibitors, though the evidence remains scant. Unlike the other TNF inhibitors, it has not been observed to cause a lupus-like syndrome.

### 3.5 Certolizumab pegol

Certolizumab pegol (Cimzia®, UCB, Inc., Smyrna, GA, USA) is approved for the treatment of moderate to severe rheumatoid arthritis, psoriatic arthritis, and Crohn's disease. Unlike fellow anti-TNF monoclonal antibodies, this agent is a polyethylene glycolated Fab fragment.

#### *3.5.1 Administration*

Certolizumab is initially administered as subcutaneous injections of 400 mg at weeks 0, 2, and 4, then continued as 400 mg injections monthly, or 200 mg injections every other week.

#### *3.5.2 Efficacy*

While certolizumab has shown efficacy in the management of systemic inflammation, limited data exist regarding its utility in uveitis at this time. A single retrospective case series of seven patients reports experience in the treatment of chronic immune-mediated uveitis (Behçet's disease, ankylosing spondylitis, psoriatic arthritis, and idiopathic retinal vasculitis) that had failed other TNF inhibitor therapy due to loss of efficacy or development of serious adverse effects. Over a mean follow-up period of 10.4 months, five of these seven patients developed quiescence with improvement in visual acuity and central macular thickness, with benefit seen as early as 1 month after initiation of certolizumab [23]. Another study reports decreased incidence of uveitis flares with certolizumab comparable to rates reported for other anti-TNF-α agents, but did not have sufficient numbers to establish statistical significance [24].

#### *3.5.3 Safety*

Existing reports on the use of certolizumab suggest risk for development of autoimmunity. It has been associated with a lupus-like syndrome, as well as bilateral panuveitis secondary to an ocular sarcoidosis-like reaction in a patient with rheumatoid arthritis and no prior history of sarcoidosis; signs and symptoms were noted to resolve following cessation of certolizumab in these cases [25, 26].

## 4. Adverse effects

### 4.1 Infections

TNF-α plays a crucial role in host immunity against infections, and correspondingly, blockade of TNF predisposes individuals to opportunistic infections, as well as reactivation of latent tuberculosis and hepatitis viruses. Patients on anti-TNF-α treatment also experience increased rates of invasive fungal infections, including histoplasmosis and coccidioidomycosis. Therefore, prior to initiating therapy, patients should be screened for active and latent tuberculosis with skin testing or an interferon gamma release assay, with a follow-up chest X-ray should these screening exams return positive. Patients who are diagnosed with tuberculosis should be treated for at least 1 month prior to initiating anti-TNF-α therapy. Hepatitis screening should also be performed before starting TNF inhibitors, with preceding hepatitis B vaccination for individuals not immune to hepatitis B, and concomitant prophylaxis against hepatitis virus reactivation during anti-TNF therapy for those with serologic evidence of hepatitis infection. Finally, pneumococcal and influenza vaccinations should also be considered. Once TNF-α inhibitors are started, live vaccines and unpasteurized milk should be avoided to reduce the risk of disseminated infection.

### 4.2 Malignancies

There is conflicting evidence in the literature regarding the risk of new as well as recurrence of prior malignancies with TNF-α therapy. Some registries have noted an increased incidence of lymphoma and melanoma in these patients, and the FDA issued a black box warning in 2008 regarding potential association between use of TNF inhibitors and development of these cancers in children and young adults. Other studies report that TNF inhibitors may accelerate diagnosis of cancer in the first year of treatment, but may not increase long-term cancer risk [27]. Evidence for this may be confounded by the number of underlying conditions and history of other immunosuppressant therapy that patients carry. Regardless, patients being considered for TNF-α blockade should be informed of this potential risk.

### 4.3 Demyelinating disease and neuropathies

TNF inhibitors have been associated with central and peripheral neuropathies, including demyelinating and vasculitic neuropathies, and the pathogenesis for this phenomenon is unknown. A number of series have reported the development of Guillain-Barre syndrome and demyelinating lesions in the central nervous system similar to those in multiple sclerosis following initiation of anti-TNF-α therapy [28, 29]. For this reason, an MRI of the brain is recommended for patients with intermediate uveitis prior to starting TNF inhibitors to rule out underlying demyelinating disease, and these agents should not be prescribed to patients with evidence of demyelinating disease. If patients carry a positive family history, the risk of developing demyelinating disease should be discussed with them before proceeding with TNF-α blockers.

### 4.4 Congestive heart failure

Reports of atherosclerosis formation, promotion of plaque rupture, hypertrophy and heart failure from contractile myocardial dysfunction have been described with anti-TNF-α blockade. The New York Heart Association (NYHA) recommends against the use of TNF inhibitors in patients with NYHA class III or IV heart failure [30]. Those patients with compensated congestive heart failure (NYHA classes I or II) should undergo a baseline evaluation and be followed closely for any signs of worsening heart failure while on anti-TNF-α therapy.

### 4.5 Induction of autoimmunity

Anti-TNF-α agents may induce autoimmunity and formation of auto-antibodies, including antinuclear, anti-DNA, and anti-cardiolipin antibodies, among others. All of the TNF inhibitors, especially etanercept, have been associated with the onset of sarcoidosis [26, 31]. A rare lupus-like syndrome has been reported with all TNF antagonists with the exception of golimumab, and most commonly with etanercept and infliximab [32]. Other autoimmune diseases that have been reported include leukocytoclastic vasculitis, interstitial lung diseases, antiphospholipid syndrome-related features, autoimmune hepatitis and uveitis [31].

### 4.6 Endogenous uveitis

Paradoxically, there are reports associating TNF inhibitors with the onset or recurrence of uveitis, particularly with etanercept [33]. The mechanism is unclear, but one speculation is that as a soluble receptor, etanercept may prolong the half-life of TNF in the eye and potentiate uveitis if the receptor-ligand complex is not cleared promptly. Compared to infliximab, etanercept also has differential effects on T-lymphocytes and does not induce apoptosis. These differences may also contribute to observations of decreased efficacy of etanercept in certain inflammatory conditions [34].

### 4.7 Infusion reactions

The most common adverse effects of TNF inhibitor therapy are hypersensitivity reactions to the drug infusion, which are felt to be related to immune-complex formation and deposition. Most reactions are characterized by cutaneous, eczema-like eruptions at the site of injection, but may also include fever, nausea and vomiting, and arthralgia. These reactions may occur immediately after administration or in a delayed fashion up to 2 weeks after treatment. Of note, infliximab has been associated with a high rate of hypersensitivity reactions in up to 22% of patients undergoing infusion, and has been reported to cause angioedema and anaphylaxis [35]. Patients are hence often pre-medicated with Benadryl and acetaminophen to prevent these reactions.

### 4.8 Pregnancy

Pregnancy outcomes for women on infliximab have been reported through the Infliximab Safety Database and the Crohn's Therapy, Resource, Evaluation and Assessment Tool (TREAT) registry, without evidence for an increased rate of miscarriages, birth complications, or fetal anomalies above that of the general pregnant population [36]. As an IgG antibody, infliximab does not cross the placenta during the first trimester, but readily crosses during the late second and third trimesters, and can subsequently persist in the infant for months after birth [37]. Therefore, based upon this and registry-reported outcomes, infliximab is generally considered safe during the first trimester and majority of the second trimester. However, it is advised that patients stop the drug during the late second or third trimester to minimize transfer to the fetus, and to avoid administering live vaccines to infants exposed to infliximab *in utero* given their increased risk for disseminated infection.

As a pegylated Fc-free agent, certolizumab does not cross the placenta in significant amounts, and is thus thought to be safer in pregnancy [38]. The largest published database on certolizumab use in pregnant women to date examined outcomes of 1137 prospectively reported pregnancies, without finding increased risk for teratogenic effects or fetal death as compared to the general population [38].

## 5. Monitoring clinical response

Once the decision has been made to proceed with TNF-α blockade, it is important to closely monitor patients for clinical response, as well as unwanted secondary effects. General routine clinical evaluation for infections, cytopenias, demyelinating disease, cancer, and cardiovascular alterations is essential, and may need to be performed in conjunction with a multidisciplinary team of specialists. Patient should also undergo serologic testing with a complete blood count and comprehensive metabolic profile every month for the first 3 months and at least every 2–4 months afterward. If testing results are abnormal, anti-TNF-α therapy should be deferred until these parameters have normalized.

The rate of nonresponse has been reported to be approximately 20% for patients initiated on infliximab therapy for uveitis [39]. Treatment response may depend on various factors, including age, location and severity of uveitis, and type of TNF-α blocker used. Genetic polymorphisms in TNF receptors and promoter regions may also impact the response to anti-TNF treatment.

Immunogenicity, in which an antigen induces an immune response after being recognized by a preexisting T-cell or B-cell receptor, may also occur and account for suboptimal response or treatment failure. This may lead to drug trough levels that are lower than expected or the appearance of serum anti-drug antibodies, which lead to drug-antibody complex formation and consequent rapid clearance of the drug. Ocular and systemic inflammation may subsequently become resistant after several months of treatment. This phenomenon is most prevalent with infliximab, in which case these antibodies are referred to as human anti-chimeric antibodies (HACA), but also occurs with use of adalimumab.

Cordero-Coma and colleagues have summarized a proposal for patients not responsive or poorly responsive to anti-TNF therapy based on other studies [40]. If a patient is deemed to have insufficient clinical response to anti-TNF-α therapy, work-up of these patients with serum drug trough and anti-drug antibody levels may be warranted to guide management. High serum drug levels correlate with clinical response and decreased risk for relapse, and dosing should be individually optimized to attain a therapeutic drug level [41]. In patients with low drug trough levels, one should consider intensifying therapy by either increasing the dosage of each treatment or the frequency of dosing (up to every 4–6 weeks for infliximab and every week for adalimumab). If patients have suboptimal clinical response despite sufficient drug trough concentration, an alternative immunosuppressant with different mode of action may be required to control disease activity. Regardless of serum drug concentration, if anti-drug antibody levels are high, one should consider either switching to an alternative TNF inhibitor and/or adding concomitant steroids or other immunosuppression. Studies have shown that the traditional approach of intensifying therapy in antibody-positive patients is inferior to switching agents, with less treatment success and increased expense and risk of adverse effects [42].

There is not yet consensus regarding the preferred mode of assessing drug and antibody levels. Several assays are available, including enzyme-linked immunosorbent assay (ELISA), radioimmunoassay, reporter gene assay, and homogeneous mobility shift assay, each with their own advantages and drawbacks. ELISA is the most readily accessible, but suffers from false-positive and false-negative results; the other modalities are more precise but logistically difficult to obtain [43].

## 6. Expert panel recommendations

In 2014, an Expert panel comprising a subcommittee of the American Uveitis Society published recommendations regarding the evidence-based use of anti-TNF-α agents [44]:

- Infliximab and adalimumab can be considered in preference to etanercept, which is associated with lower rates of treatment success.

- Infliximab and adalimumab can be considered first-line for treatment of ocular manifestations of Behçet's disease.

- Infliximab and adalimumab can be considered second-line for uveitis associated with juvenile arthritis.

- Infliximab and adalimumab can be considered potential second-line treatments for severe ocular inflammatory conditions, including posterior or panuveitis, severe uveitis associated with seronegative spondyloarthropathy, and scleritis in patients who have failed or are not candidates for antimetabolites or calcineurin inhibitors.

## 7. Conclusions and future directions

Tumor necrosis factor alpha inhibitors are mainstay treatments for several systemic immune-mediated conditions, including rheumatoid arthritis, juvenile arthritis, ankylosing spondylitis, inflammatory bowel disease, and psoriatic arthritis, and serve as an important pillar of immunomodulatory therapy in the treatment of uveitis. Infliximab and adalimumab have both been shown to be successful at controlling ocular inflammation, particularly that related to Behçet's disease and juvenile arthritis. However, serious potential side effects, such as risk for opportunistic infections, reactivation of latent tuberculosis, and malignancy, may limit their use in uveitis. Further studies of the newer agents, golimumab and certolizumab, are warranted to establish their efficacy in uveitis, but early data regarding their safety have been promising, and they may represent future additional treatment options within this class.

Future directions for anti-TNF therapy include further studies of the significance of intravitreal formulations, as well as the development of biosimilars that may represent comparable and more affordable options to the traditional TNF antagonists. Intravitreal therapy with anti-TNF agents has been utilized and evaluated in very few studies with small sample sizes. The results have been variable and whether local therapy to the eye with these agents is safe and effective remains to be seen [45–48]. Biosimilars, defined by the World Health Organization as a biotherapeutic product which is similar in terms of quality, safety, and efficacy to an already licensed reference biotherapeutic product, provide potential economic alternatives to the current TNF-α agents. Despite the effectiveness and relatively rapid action of TNF inhibitors, the high cost may hinder accessibility to these drugs for some patients. A 2016 systematic review of 19 observational studies and clinical trials comparing biosimilar TNF-α inhibitors concluded that evidence supports the efficacy and safety of these agents [49]. The most notable existing biosimilar within this class is infliximab-dyyb, which exhibits similar qualities to the original product infliximab, and is currently available in many countries and was approved by the FDA in 2016. Several others are in development or already licensed for use outside the United States. As biosimilars become available, they may improve patient accessibility to these drugs for disabling disease.

## Acknowledgements

Funding was provided by an unrestricted departmental grant from Research to Prevent Blindness (all authors), P30 EY00179 (all authors), and National Institute of Health/National Eye Institute K12 grant EY021475 (AMLC).

## Conflict of interest

The authors have no conflicts of interest.

## Author details

Judy L. Chen, Ann-Marie Lobo-Chan, Robison Vernon Paul Chan and Pooja Bhat*
Illinois Eye and Ear Infirmary, University of Illinois at Chicago, Chicago, Illinois, USA

*Address all correspondence to: pbhat@uic.edu

## References

[1] Carswell EA, Old LJ, Kassel RL, et al. An endotoxin-induced serum factor that causes necrosis of tumors. Proceedings of the National Academy of Sciences of the United States of America. 1975;**72**(9):3666-3670. DOI: 10.1073/pnas.72.9.3666

[2] Tracey D, Klareskog L, Sasso EH, et al. Tumor necrosis factor antagonist mechanisms of action: A comprehensive review. Pharmacology & Therapeutics. 2008;**117**:244-279. DOI: 10.1016/j.pharmthera.2007.10.001

[3] Ye LL, Wei XS, Zhang M, et al. The significance of tumor necrosis factor receptor type II in CD8+ regulatory T cells and CD8+ effector T cells. Frontiers in Immunology. 2018;**9**:583. DOI: 10.3389/fimmu.2018.00583

[4] Ticha O, Moos L, Wajant H, et al. Expression of tumor necrosis factor receptor 2 characterizes TLR9-drive formation of interleukin-10-producing B cells. Frontiers in Immunology. 2018;**8**:1951. DOI: 10.3389/fimmu.2017.01951

[5] Spoettl T, Hausmann M, Klebl F, et al. Serum soluble TNF receptor I and II levels correlate with disease activity in IBD patients. Inflammatory Bowel Diseases. 2007;**13**(6):727-732. DOI: 10.1002/ibd.20107

[6] Busch M, Bauer D, Hennig M, et al. Effects of systemic and intravitreal TNF-alpha inhibition in experimental autoimmune uveoretinitis. Investigative Ophthalmology & Visual Science. 2013;**54**:39-46. DOI: 10.1167/iovs.12-10138

[7] Weir N, Athwal D, Brown D, et al. A new generation of high-affinity humanized PEGylated Fab+ fragment anti-tumor necrosis factor-(alpha) monoclonal antibodies. Therapy. 2006;**3**:535-545. DOI: 10.2217/14750708.3.4.535

[8] Heiligenhaus A, Michels H, Schumacher C, et al. Evidence-based, interdisciplinary guidelines for anti-inflammatory treatment of uveitis associated with juvenile idiopathic arthritis. Rheumatology International. 2012;**32**(5):1121-1133. DOI: 10.1007/s00296-011-2126-1

[9] Galor A, Perez VL, Hammel JP, et al. Differential effectiveness of etanercept and infliximab in the treatment of ocular inflammation. Ophthalmology. 2006;**113**(12):2317-2323. DOI: 10.1016/j.ophtha.2006.04.038

[10] Lim LL, Fraunfelder FW, Rosenbaum JT. Do tumor necrosis factor inhibitors cause uveitis? A registry-based study. Arthritis and Rheumatism. 2007;**56**(10):3248-3252. DOI: 10.1002/art.22918

[11] Van Dartel SA, Fransen J, Kierit W, et al. Difference in the risk of serious infections in patients with rheumatoid arthritis treated with adalimumab, infliximab and etanercept: Results from the Dutch Rheumatoid Arthritis Monitoring (DREAM) registry. Annals of the Rheumatic Diseases. 2013;**72**(6):895-900. DOI: 10.1136/annrheumdis-2012-201338

[12] Tambralli A, Beukelman T, Weiser P, et al. High doses of infliximab in the management of juvenile idiopathic arthritis. The Journal of Rheumatology. 2013;**40**(10):1749-1755. DOI: 10.3899/jrheum.130133

[13] Markomichelakis N, Delicha E, Masselos S, et al. A single infliximab infusion vs corticosteroids for acute panuveitis attacks in Behcet's disease: A comparative 4-week study. Rheumatology (Oxford). 2011;**50**(3):593-597. DOI: 10.1093/rheumatology/keq366

[14] Tabbara KF, Al-Hemidan AI. Infliximab effects compared

to conventional therapy in the management of retinal vasculitis in Behcet's disease. American Journal of Ophthalmology. 2008;**146**(6):845-850 e1. DOI: 10.1016/j.ajo.2008.09.010

[15] Ardoin SP, Kredich D, Rabinovich E, et al. Infliximab to treat chronic noninfectious uveitis in children: A retrospective case series with long-term follow-up. American Journal of Ophthalmology. 2007;**144**(6):844-849. DOI: 10.1016/j.ajo.2007.08.018

[16] Schaap-Fogler M, Amer R, Friling R, et al. Anti-TNF-α agents for refractory cystoid macular edema associated with noninfectious uveitis. Graefe's Archive for Clinical and Experimental Ophthalmology. 2014;**252**:633-640. DOI: 10.1007/s00417-013-2552-8

[17] Adán A, Sanmartí R, Burés, et al. Successful treatment with infliximab in a patient with diffuse subretinal fibrosis syndrome. American Journal of Ophthalmology. 2007;**143**(3):533-534. DOI: 10.1016/j.ajo.2006.10.047

[18] Suhler EB, Smith JR, Wertheim MS, et al. A prospective trial of infliximab therapy for refractory uveitis: Preliminary safety and efficacy outcomes. Archives of Ophthalmology. 2005;**123**(7):903-912. DOI: 10.1001/archopht.123.7.903

[19] Jaffe GJ, Dick AD, Brézin AP, et al. Adalimumab in patients with active noninfectious uveitis. NEJM. 2016;**375**:932-943. DOI: 10.1056/NEJMoa1509852

[20] Calleja S, Cordero-Coma M, Rodriguez E, et al. Adalimumab specifically induces CD3(+) CD4(+) CD25(high) Foxp3(+) CD127(−) T-regulatory cells and decreases vascular endothelial growth factor plasma levels in refractory immune-mediated uveitis: A non-randomized pilot intervention study. Eye (London, England). 2012;**26**(3):468-477. DOI: 10.1038/eye.2011.320

[21] Miserocchi E, Modorati G, Pontikaki I, et al. Long-term treatment with golimumab for severe uveitis. Ocular Immunology and Inflammation. 2014;**22**(2):90-95. DOI: 10.3109/09273948.2013.844265

[22] Fabiani C, Sota J, Rigante D, et al. Rapid and sustained efficacy of golimumab in the treatment of multirefractory uveitis associated with Behçet's disease. Ocular Immunology and Inflammation. 2017;**5**:1-6. DOI: 10.1080/09273948.2017.1351573

[23] Llorenç V, Mesquida M, Sainz de la Maza M, et al. Certolizumab pegol, a new anti-TNF-α in the armamentarium against ocular inflammation. Ocular Immunology and Inflammation. 2016;**24**(2):167-172. DOI: 10.3109/09273948.2014.967779

[24] Rudwaleit M, Rosenbaum JT, Landewé R, et al. Observed incidence of uveitis following certolizumab pegol treatment in patients with axial spondyloarthritis. Arthritis Care & Research (Hoboken). 2016;**68**(6):838-844. DOI: 10.1002/acr.22848

[25] Mudduluru BM, Shah S, Shamah S, et al. TNF-alpha antagonist induced lupus on three different agents. Postgraduate Medicine. 2017;**129**(2):304-306. DOI: 10.1080/00325481.2017.1249266

[26] Moisseiev E, Shulman S. Certolizumab-induced uveitis: A case report and review of the literature. Case Reports in Ophthalmology. 2014;**5**(1):54-59. DOI: 10.1159/000358324

[27] Kempen JH, Gangaputra S, Daniel E, et al. Long-term risk of malignancy among patients treated with immunosuppressive agents for ocular inflammation: A critical assessment of the evidence. American Journal of Ophthalmology. 2008;**146**(6):802-812. e1. DOI: 10.1016/j.ajo.2008.04.035

[28] Lozeron P, Denier C, Lacroix C, et al. Long-term course of demyelinating neuropathies occurring during tumor necrosis factor-alpha-blocker therapy. Archives of Neurology. 2009;**66**(4):490-497. DOI: 10.1001/archneurol.2009.11

[29] Robinson WH, Genovese MC, Moreland LW. Demyelinating and neurologic events reported in association with tumor necrosis factor alpha antagonism: By what mechanisms could tumor necrosis factor alpha antagonists improve rheumatoid arthritis but exacerbate multiple sclerosis? Arthritis and Rheumatism. 2001;**44**(9):1977-1983. DOI: 10.1002/1529-0131(200109)44:9<1977::AID-ART345>3.0.CO:2-6

[30] Chung ES, Packer M, Lo KH, et al. Randomized, double-blind, placebo-controlled, pilot trial of infliximab, a chimeric monoclonal antibody to tumor necrosis factor-α, in patients with moderate-to-severe heart failure: Results of the anti-TNF therapy against congestive heart failure (ATTACH) trial. Circulation. 2003;**107**(25):3133-3140. DOI: 10.1161/01.CIR.0000077913.60364.D2

[31] Ramos-Casals M, Brito-Zerón P, Soto MJ, et al. Autoimmune diseases induced by TNF-targeted therapies. Best Practice & Research. Clinical Rheumatology. 2008;**22**(5):847-861. DOI: 10.1016/j.berh.2008.09.008

[32] Williams VL, Cohen PR. TNF alpha antagonist-induced lupus-like syndrome: Report and review of the literature with implications for treatment with alternative TNF alpha antagonists. International Journal of Dermatology. 2011;**50**(5):619-625. DOI: 10.1111/j.1365-4632.2011.04871.x

[33] Kakkassery V, Mergler S, Pleyer U. Anti-TNF-α treatment: A possible promoter in endogenous uveitis? Observational report on six patients: Occurrence of uveitis following etanercept treatment. Current Eye Research. 2010;**35**(8):751-756. DOI: 10.3109/02713683.2010.486520

[34] Sieper J, Van Den Brande J. Diverse effects of infliximab and etanercept on T lymphocytes. Seminars in Arthritis and Rheumatism. 2005;**34**(5 Suppl 1):23-27. DOI: 10.1016/j.semarthrit.2005.01.006

[35] Puxeddu I, Giori L, Rocchi V, et al. Hypersensitivity reactions during treatment with infliximab, etanercept, and adalimumab. Annals of Allergy, Asthma & Immunology. 2012;**108**(2):123-124. DOI: 10.1016/j.anal.2011.11.004

[36] Lichtenstein GR, Feagan BG, Mahadevan U, et al. Pregnancy outcomes reported during the 13-year TREAT registry: A descriptive report. The American Journal of Gastroenterology. 2018;**113**(11):1678-1688. DOI: 10.1038/s41395-018-0202-9

[37] Djokanovic N, Klieger-Grossmann C, Pupco A, et al. Safety of infliximab use during pregnancy. Reproductive Toxicology. 2011;**32**(1):93-97. DOI: 10.1016/j.reprotox.2011.05.009

[38] Clowse MEB, Scheuerle AE, Chambers C, et al. Pregnancy outcomes after exposure to certolizumab pegol: Updated results from a pharmacovigilance safety database. Arthritis & Rhematology. 2018;**70**(9):1399-1407. DOI: 10.1002/art.40508

[39] Kruh JN, Yang P, Suelves AM, et al. Infliximab for the treatment of refractory noninfectious uveitis: A study of 88 patients with long-term follow-up. Ophthalmology. 2014;**121**:358-364. DOI: 10.1016/j.ophtha.2013.07.019

[40] Cordero-Coma M, Sobrin L. Anti-tumor necrosis factor-α therapy in uveitis. Survey of Ophthalmology. 2015;**60**(6):575-589. DOI: 10.1016/j.survophthal.2015.06.004

[41] Colombel JF, Feagan BG, Sandborn WJ, et al. Therapeutic drug monitoring of biologics for inflammatory bowel disease. Inflammatory Bowel Diseases. 2012;**18**:349-358. DOI: 10.1002/ibd.21831

[42] Mok CC, Tsai WC, Chen DY, et al. Immunogenicity of anti-TNF biologic agents in the treatment of rheumatoid arthritis. Expert Opinion on Biological Therapy. 2016;**16**(2):201-211. DOI: 10.1517/14712598.2016.1118457

[43] Cao F, Cao H, Cao X. A review of six methods for monitoring infliximab concentrations and antibodies to infliximab. International Journal of Clinical Pharmacology and Therapeutics. 2017;**55**(7):571-580. DOI: 10.5414/CP202945

[44] Levy-Clarke G, Jabs DA, Read RW, Rosenbaum JT, Vitale A, Van Gelder RN. Expert panel recommendations for the use of anti-tumor necrosis factor biologic agents in patients with ocular inflammatory disorders. Ophthalmology. 2014;**121**(3):785-796. DOI: 10.1016/j.ophtha.2013.09.048

[45] Androudi S, Tsironi E, Kalogeropoulos C, et al. Intravitreal adalimumab for refractory uveitis-related macular edema. Ophthalmology. 2010;**117**(8):1612-1616. DOI: 10.1016/j.ophtha.2009.12.011

[46] Farvardin M, Afarid M, Shahrzad S. Long-term effects of intravitreal infliximab for treatment of sight-threatening chronic noninfectious uveitis. Journal of Ocular Pharmacology and Therapeutics. 2012;**28**(6):628-631. DOI: 10.1089/jop.2011.0199

[47] Markomichelakis N, Delicha E, Masselos S, et al. Intravitreal infliximab for sight-threatening relapsing uveitis in Behçet disease: A pilot study in 15 patients. American Journal of Ophthalmology. 2012;**154**(3):534, 41.e1. DOI: 10.1016/j.ajo.2012.03.035

[48] Hamza MM, Macky TA, Sidky MK, et al. Intravitreal infliximab in refractory uveitis in Behçet's disease: A safety and efficacy clinical study. Retina. 2016;**36**(12):2399-2408. DOI: 10.1097/IAE.0000000000001109

[49] Blair HA, Deeks ED. Infliximab biosimilar (CT-P13; Infliximab-dyyb): A review in autoimmune inflammatory diseases. BioDrugs. 2016;**30**(5):469-480. DOI: 10.1007/s40259-016-0193-2